T0178823

Myasthenia in Children

Clinics in Developmental Medicine

Myasthenia in Children

Edited by

Sandeep Jayawant

Consultant in Paediatric Neurology,
Oxford Childrens Hospital;
Honorary Senior Clinical Lecturer,
University of Oxford, Oxford, UK

2020
Mac Keith Press

© 2020 Mac Keith Press

Managing Director: Ann-Marie Halligan
Senior Publishing Manager: Sally Wilkinson
Publishing Co-ordinator: Lucy White
Project Management: Riverside Publishing Solutions Ltd

First published in this edition in 2019 by Mac Keith Press
2nd Floor, Rankin Building, 139–143 Bermondsey Street, London, SE1 3UW

British Library Cataloguing-in-Publication data
A catalogue record for this book is available from the British Library

Cover designer: Marten Sealby

ISBN: 978-1-911612-29-2

Typeset by Riverside Publishing Solutions Ltd

Printed by Jellyfish Solutions Ltd

Dedication

I started my book with great encouragement from my wife Girija, my partner, my strength and my leading light. Through the process of writing this book she was suddenly taken away from me last year. Her love and cherished memories and my children Saahil and Saania have given me the strength to carry on with this work. I want to dedicate this book to my wife Girija Jayawant (1971–2018).

Sandeep Jayawant

Contents

Author Appointments

David Beeson
Professor in Molecular Neurosciences, NDCN University of Oxford, Weatherall Institute of Molecular Medicine, The John Radcliffe Hospital, Oxford, UK

Samyami Chowdhury
Specialist Registrar in Paediatric Neurology, Oxford Childrens Hospital, Oxford, UK

David Hilton-Jones
Consultant in Neurology, Nuffield Department of Neurological Sciences, University of Oxford, Oxford, UK

Andrew Ives
Consultant in Paediatric Respiratory Medicine, Oxford Childrens Hospital, Oxford, UK

Sandeep Jayawant
Consultant in Paediatric Neurology, Oxford Childrens Hospital; Honorary Senior Clinical Lecturer, University of Oxford, Oxford, UK

Heinz Jungbluth
Professor of Paediatric Neurology, Kings College London; Consultant Paediatric Neurologist Evelina Children's Hospital, Guy's & St Thomas' NHS Foundation Trust, London, UK

Nancy L Kuntz
Professor in Pediatrics and Neurology, Northwestern Feinberg School of Medicine; Attending Neurologist, Ann and Robert H. Lurie Children's Hospital, Chicago, Illinois, USA

Pinki Munot
Consultant in Paediatric Neurology, Great Ormond Street Hospital, London, UK

Jacqueline Palace
Consultant in Neurology, and Associate Professor, Nuffield Department of Neurological Sciences, University of Oxford, Oxford, UK

Jeremy Parr
Professor of Paediatric Neurodisability, Great North Children's Hospital, Newcastle upon Tyne NHS Foundation Trust; Institute of Neuroscience, Newcastle University, Newcastle, UK

Matthew Pitt
Consultant in Clinical Neurophysiology, Great Ormond Street Hospital, London, UK

Sithara Ramdas
Consultant in Paediatric Neurology, Oxford Childrens Hospital, Oxford, UK

Hayley Ramjattan
Specialist Paediatric Neuromuscular Physiotherapist (Congenital Myasthenia Service), Oxford Childrens Hospital, Oxford, UK

Vamshi K Rao
Assistant Professor in Pediatrics, Northwestern University; Ann & Robert H. Lurie Children's Hospital, Chicago, Illinois, USA

Stephanie Robb
Consultant in Paediatric Neurology, Great Ormond Street Hospital, London, UK

Pedro M Rodríguez Cruz   Clinical Research Fellow, Weatherall Institute of Molecular Medicine, Nuffield Department of Clinical Neurosciences, University of Oxford, Oxford, UK

Adam Webster   Young Adult Service User, Congenital Myasthenia Service, Cardiff, Wales, UK

Gordon Webster   Research Associate, School of Biosciences, Cardiff University, Wales, UK

James Webster   Young Adult Service User, Congenital Myasthenia Service, Cardiff, Wales, UK

Kerry Webster   Webster Family (Clients of Congenital Myasthenia Service), Cardiff, Wales, UK

Foreword

This excellent book is the product of a stellar authorship including international researchers, experienced clinicians and an affected family.

Clear, succinct, practical and focussed, it will be a valuable resource to everyone from the general paediatrician with an affected patient, through neurophysiologists, geneticists, paediatric respirologists and physiotherapists with a commitment to one or more children with myasthenia, to paediatric neurologists in training and in practice.

The book is rationally organised into a sequence of 12 chapters covering the structure and physiology of the neuromuscular junction, its neurophysiological investigation, the types of transmission disorder and their clinical symptomatology, epidemiology, the auto-immune myasthenias, the congenital myasthenias, drug (and other) treatment, neuromuscular transmission defects associated with other disorders of nerve and muscle, respiratory assessment and management, physio- and occupational therapy and the paediatric to adult transition process. The final chapter is a compelling and instructive description of the experience of congenital myasthenia from an affected family.

Tables and diagrams are well-spaced and illuminating. They include, for example, an excellent summary of the characteristic clinical features and treatment options for the auto-immune childhood myasthenias (see Table 5.1, p 41) followed later in the same chapter by an accessible flow-chart of the potential sequences of intervention in this group (see Figure 5.1, p 44). In a later chapter, there is an excellent schematic representation of the neuromuscular junction illustrating the principle molecules involved in congenital myasthenia. A masterly table in the seventh chapter summarises the relevant drug treatments (and contraindications) for the individual congenital myasthenic syndromes (see Table 7.1, p 70).

The book ends with an inspiring, vivid, informative and practical account of living with myasthenia by a family with three affected members. It is essential reading for involved professionals and for many patients. It includes a wide-ranging set of useful web-sites.

Each chapter ends with a robust and relevant reference list.

The key qualities of this superb book are its combination of comprehensiveness, clarity and succinctness. Every paediatric neurologist should have a copy as should every paediatric, neonatal, genetics and neurophysiology library. Any clinician who finds themselves responsible for any aspect of care for this challenging group of conditions will find it an essential resource. I recommend it unreservedly.

Dr Michael Pike MA, MD, FRCPCH
Honorary Consultant Paediatric Neurologist
Oxford Children's Hospital

Preface

Myasthenia is a rare disorder in children. It can result from an autoimmune disorder or a genetic mutation. There have been significant developments in identification and treatment of myasthenia in recent years. Congenital Myasthenic Syndromes are expanding with their unique clinical phenotypes. There is no guideline on diagnosis or treatment of this rare disorder. The authors have between them a number of years' experience of diagnosing and managing this rare condition which can result in significant morbidity and mortality. Oxford is the National Centre for Congenital Myasthenic Syndromes in the United Kingdom. This book brings together all this experience and practical suggestions from different authors and experts in this field across Europe and North America. This book gives clinicians guidance on diagnosing and managing these rare conditions appropriately and promptly. Sections on therapy set out clear treatment guidelines. There are chapters on supportive management such as physiotherapy, occupational therapy and respiratory management which are equally important in improving quality of life for these children and their families. A patient's perspective makes this a useful resource for children and their families and offers solutions to some of their day to day issues in work, school and at home. I hope this book will be of interest to clinicians, patients, their families and therapist colleagues treating these rare conditions for which there is little practical advice available even on the internet.

This leaves me to thank all my colleagues and collaborators in this exercise to bring the readership a broad and in-depth overview of this rare childhood condition. Without much written material available on this condition they have done their absolute best to bring all their knowledge and experience to you. My sincere thanks to them.

Sandeep Jayawant
June 2019

Acknowledgements

I would like to thank Mac Keith Press who were so supportive, encouraging and helpful at every stage of the process. I would like to thank my collaborators and contributors to this book, especially the Webster family. My special thanks to Professor Beeson and the late Professor Newsom-Davies who introduced me to the world of Congenital Myasthenia and fired my interest in the subject and also to the entire Oxford CMS Service. My special thanks to my colleagues and teachers Dr Mike Pike and Dr Tony McShane who have inspired me to enjoy Paediatric Neurology.

Sandeep Jayawant

The Neuromuscular Junction

Pedro M Rodríguez Cruz and David Beeson

The neuromuscular junction (NMJ) is a highly specialised synapse between a motor neuron and a muscle fibre, which is essential for neuromuscular transmission. In this chapter, the most fundamental aspects of the NMJ organisation, structure and physiology biology, and physiology will be reviewed. This will provide the background to understanding the physiopathology and clinical manifestations of myasthenic disorders, either autoimmune (myasthenia gravis; MG) or genetic (congenital myasthenic syndromes; CMS).

ORGANISATION OF THE NEUROMUSCULAR JUNCTION

NMJs are very small structures (~20μm) compared to the length of the muscle fibres they innervate. Typically, each skeletal muscle fibre has a single NMJ where the motor axon joins the muscle. The most common classification divides the NMJ into a presynaptic terminal, a postsynaptic muscle membrane and the space that lies between, called the synaptic cleft (Fig. 1.1). The classic morphology of the NMJ in murine animal models is described as a pretzel-shaped structure. However, human NMJs are typically smaller, less complex, and more fragmented than the NMJs studied in murine animal models (Jones et al. 2017), although human NMJs exhibit a higher degree of folding than the NMJs of any other species (Slater 2017).

Presynaptic Terminal

Motor nerves travel from the spinal cord to skeletal muscles where they divide into terminal branches and subsequently form synaptic boutons that contact the muscle surface (Desaki and Uehara 1981). Synaptic buttons are small protuberances found at the terminal end of motor axons. They are filled with synaptic vesicles containing the neurotransmitter acetylcholine (ACh) ready for vesicle exocytosis upon the arrival of an action potential (Figs. 1.1 and 1.2). The nerve terminal has a complex machinery in place to allow the synthesis, exocytosis and recycling of synaptic vesicles (Lai et al. 2017). Terminal Schwann cells cover the NMJ although their role in synapse formation and maintenance is still unclear (Feng and Ko 2008).

Synaptic Cleft

The synaptic cleft is the space between the presynaptic nerve terminal and the postsynaptic muscle membrane, which is filled with a specialised form of extracellular matrix called the synaptic basal lamina (Sanes 2003). This matrix is crucial for the alignment, organisation and structural integrity of the NMJ. The main components of the basal lamina include laminins, collagens, heparan sulfate proteoglycans (muscle agrin and perlecan) and nidogens (Shi et al. 2012). It should be noted that the enzyme acetylcholinesterase (AChE), which terminates synaptic transmission by breaking down acetylcholine, is attached to the basal lamina by a collagenic tail (Ohno et al. 1998).

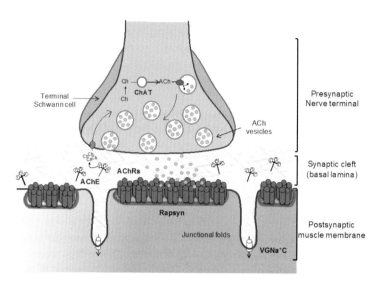

Figure 1.1   Schematic representation of the neuromuscular junction. The NMJ is divided into three different compartments. The presynaptic nerve terminal is responsible for the synthesis (ChAT) and recycling of acetylcholine and the exocytosis of synaptic vesicles. The synaptic cleft contains a specialised form of extracellular matrix called basal lamina that is essential for the structural integrity of the NMJ. This the location of the enzyme AChE, which breaks down ACh into Ch. At the postsynaptic muscle compartment, the AChRs are densely clustered at the top of the junctional folds forming a network with the intracellular anchoring protein rapsyn that stabilises AChRs (Zuber and Unwin 2013). VGNa+C located at the bottom of the junctional folds are essential in the generation and propagation of action potentials. ACh, acetylcholine; AChE, acetylcholinesterase; AChR, acetylcholine receptor; Ch, choline; ChAT, choline acetyltransferase; NMJ, neuromuscular junction; VGNa+C, voltage-gated sodium channel. A colour version of this figure can be seen in the plate section.

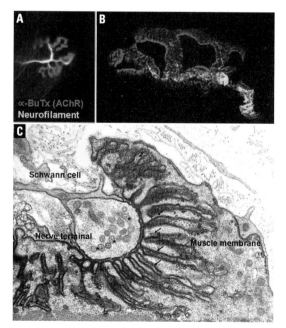

Figure 1.2   Fluorescence and electron microscopy images of the neuromuscular junction. A Fluorescence microscopy image of the NMJ showing the nerve terminal (green) innervating the muscle endplate (red) stained with fluorescently conjugated α-bungarotoxin that binds to the AChRs. **B** Super-resolution confocal microscopy image of the NMJ showing the postsynaptic muscle membrane and the junctional folds at the top of which AChRs are concentrated (image provided by Dr J. Cheung). **C** Electron microscopy image of the NMJ. The presynaptic nerve terminal is filled with synaptic vesicles containing acetylcholine (*). The postsynaptic muscle membrane exhibits a high degree of folding which extends into the muscle sarcoplasm (arrows) in order to increase the total endplate surface. The NMJ is covered by terminal Schwann cells. AChR, acetylcholine receptor; NMJ, neuromuscular junction. Adapted from Slater (2017) with permission. A colour version of this figure can be seen in the plate section.

Postsynaptic Muscle Membrane

The postsynaptic muscle membrane is a specialised structure with a high degree of folding, as shown by electron microscopy studies (De Harven and Coers 1959) (Fig. 1.2). Motor nerve terminals are embedded in the muscle in a gutter or primary cleft. Furthermore, there are a series of invaginations of the muscle membrane that extend into the sarcoplasm which are called secondary junctional folds; these increase the overall surface of the postsynaptic membrane. The acetylcholine receptors (AChRs) are clustered at high density on the crest of these folds. At the bottoms of the folds, voltage-gated Na^+ channels (VGNa$^+$C) are concentrated to facilitate the excitability of the postsynaptic membrane.

NEUROMUSCULAR JUNCTION DEVELOPMENT, MATURATION AND MAINTENANCE

During development, the axons of motor neurons are guided to innervate skeletal muscles through a process that is still not fully understood (Wu et al. 2010). In particular it is unclear whether motor neurons or muscles fibres determine the exact location of the muscle endplate. In vivo studies in mice have shown that primitive AChRs are prepatterned in the central region of the muscle (Fig. 1.3) prior to the arrival of the motor axon (Lin et al. 2001).

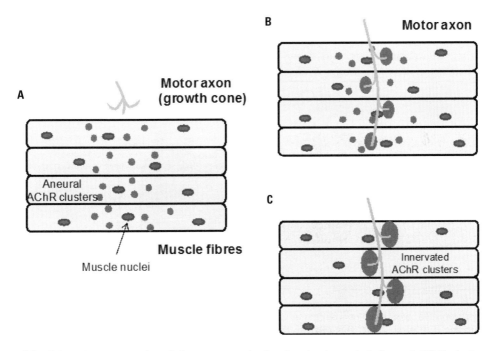

Figure 1.3   Schematic representation of the neuromuscular junction development. A Aneural AChR clusters are prepatterned in the midbelly of the muscle fibres prior to the arrival of the nerve terminal. **B** Upon innervation of the prepatterned clusters in the synaptic region, they become enlarged while aneural clusters located in the extrasynaptic region disappear. **C** As a result, AChR clusters are concentrated at a high density in the area underneath the nerve terminal maximising the efficiency of neuromuscular transmission. AChR, acetylcholine receptor. Adapted from Lin et al. (2001) with permission from Springer Nature. A colour version of this figure can be seen in the plate section.

It has been shown that this phenomenon also occurs in mutant animals lacking motor nerves, which suggests that prepatterning is nerve-independent (Yang et al. 2001). Subsequently, when the motor neurons innervate some of the prepatterned AChR clusters these become enlarged, while aneural AChR clusters tend to disappear. It is thought that neuronal agrin (McMahan 1990), a motor neuron-secreted proteoglycan that binds to the postsynaptic muscle membrane, drives the process by activating the LRP4-MuSK-DOK7 pathway which is crucial for the clustering of AChRs underneath the nerve terminal (Fig. 1.4).

On the other hand, aneural clusters not stabilised by agrin signalling are dispersed by a negative signal. This pathway is believed to be driven by the release of acetylcholine by the nerve terminal through a cyclin-dependent kinase 5 (CdK5) mechanism (Lin et al. 2005) linked to the interaction of the intracellular anchoring protein rapsyn and the calcium-dependent protease calpain (Chen et al. 2007).

Disruption of MuSK signalling postnatally is also deleterious for the NMJ structure and function (Barik et al. 2014; Tezuka et al. 2014). Therefore, these mechanisms are not only crucial for the development and maturation of the NMJ but for its maintenance during adulthood. Autoantibodies against MuSK cause autoimmune MuSK myasthenia gravis (Hoch et al. 2001). On the other hand, mutations within the clustering pathway, especially in the *DOK7* gene, are responsible for a meaningful proportion of congenital myasthenic syndromes (Beeson et al. 2006).

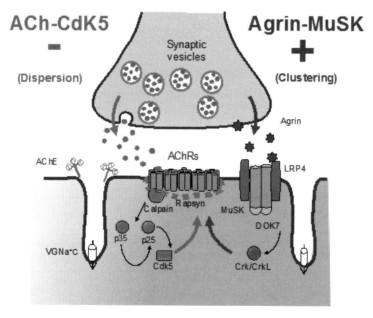

Figure 1.4   Schematic representation the neuromuscular junction and the acetylcholine receptor clustering and dispersal pathways. Upon the release of agrin by the nerve terminal, agrin binds to LRP4 resulting in MuSK dimerisation and activation (Kim et al. 2008). This leads to the recruitment of DOK7 (Okada et al. 2006), a muscle-specific cytoplas- mic adaptor of MuSK that further stimulates MuSK activation propagating the signal downstream which results in the clustering of the AChRs by the cytoplasmic anchoring protein rapsyn. By contrast, ACh is believed to disperse AChR clusters through a cyclin-dependent kinase (CdK5) mechanism linked to the interaction of rapsyn and the calcium-dependent protease calpain (Chen et al. 2007). Calpain activity promotes the cleavage of p35 to p25 (Patrick et al. 1999), an activator of CdK5. Rapsyn is believed to stabilise AChR clusters by suppressing calpain activity. ACh, acetylcholine; AChR, acetylcholine receptor; LRP4, low-density lipoprotein receptor 4; MuSK, muscle-specific kinase; VGNa+C, voltage-gated Na+ channel. Adapted from Rodriguez Cruz et al. (2018) with permission. A colour version of this figure can be seen in the plate section.

Schwann cells

Schwann cells are the main glial cells of the peripheral nervous system (PNS) and can be subdivided into two types: myelinating and non-myelinating. In contrast to myelinating Schwann cells, which ensheath axons to allow efficient electrical impulse propagation, significantly less is known about non-myelinating Schwann cells. There are three types of non-myelinating Schwann cells: Remak SCs, specialised sensory transducers (such as Pacinian corpuscles), and tSCs, which differ in structure and location. tSCs (also known as perisynaptic Schwann cells or teloglia), are non-myelinating Schwann cells that reside at the NMJ and play a vital role in the growth and maintenance of the synapse. They are integral contributors to NMJ function and recovery, and show numerous pathological changes. An improved understanding of tSCs may help decipher the pathogenesis of disease and provide new therapeutic targets for the many patients who suffer from peripheral nerve injuries and neuromuscular diseases (Santosa et al. 2018). A study by Barik et al. (2016) also highlights that Schwann cells are not only required for NMJ formation, but also necessary for its maintenance; and postsynaptic function and structure appear to be more sensitive to Schwann cell ablation.

THE PHYSIOLOGY OF NEUROMUSCULAR TRANSMISSION

Synthesis and recycling of acetylcholine

Acetylcholine is synthesised by the enzyme choline acetyltransferase (ChAT) (Nachmansohn and Machado 1943) from acetyl coenzyme A (AcCoA) and choline. Subsequently, acetylcholine is packed into synaptic vesicles thanks to the vesicular acetylcholine transporter (VAChT) (Roghani et al. 1994). Pools of synaptic vesicles accumulate in the presynaptic terminal near release sites, termed active zones (Südhof 2012), ready to be released upon the arrival of an action potential (Fig. 1.5). The necessary choline for the synthesis of

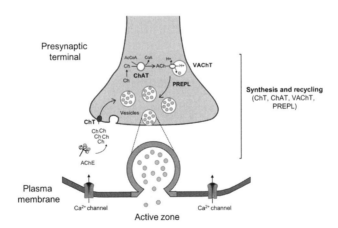

Figure 1.5   **Schematic representation of the nerve terminal and the main molecules involved in the synthesis and recycling of acetylcholine.** In the synaptic cleft, AChE breaks down acetylcholine (ACh) into acetate and Ch, which is uptaken by the ChT to the presynaptic terminal. The enzyme ChAT catalyses the synthesis of ACh from AcCoA and choline, and the vesicular acetylcholine transporter VAChT loads ACh into synaptic vesicles. *PREPL* encodes a protein thought to be involved in the trafficking of VAChT. Adapted from Ma et al. (2013). AcCoA, acetyl coenzyme A; ACh, acetylcholine; AChE, acetylcholinesterase; AChR, acetylcholine receptor; Ch, choline; ChAT, choline acetyltransferase; ChT, sodium-dependent high-affinity choline transporter 1; NMJ, neuromuscular junction; VAChT, vesicular acetylcholine transporter; VGNa+C, voltage-gated sodium channel. A colour version of this figure can be seen in the plate section.

acetylcholine is uptaken from the synaptic cleft thanks to the high-affinity choline transporter 1 (ChT) after breakdown of acetylcholine. Mutations in the genes encoding ChAT, VAChT and ChT result in a group of congenital myasthenic syndromes characterised by episodic apnoeas (Ohno et al. 2001; Bauché et al. 2016). Antibodies against the voltage-gated calcium channels located in the presynaptic terminal are responsible for Lambert–Eaton myasthenic syndrome (LEMS) (Eaton and Lambert 1957).

Release of Synaptic Vesicles at the Presynaptic Terminal

Synaptic vesicles loaded with ACh need to dock and be primed near release sites, termed active zones (Südhof 2012). Upon the arrival of an action potential, voltage-dependent Ca^{2+} channels open and the influx of Ca^{2+} cause the fusion of vesicles to the plasma membrane through the Soluble N-ethylmaleimide-sensitive factor Attachment protein REceptor (SNARE) complex and associated proteins (Baker and Hughson 2016) (Fig. 6).

Binding of Acetylcholine to the Acetylcholine Receptor

The adult nicotinic AChR is a pentameric complex composed of four different transmembrane subunits (2 α, β, δ and ε–subunits) (Karlin 2002). Acetylcholine released by the nerve terminal binds to the

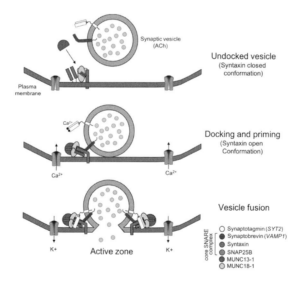

Figure 1.6   Schematic representation of synaptic vesicles at the active zones of presynaptic terminals. The influx of Ca^{2+} following an action potential causes synaptic vesicles to fuse to the plasma membrane through SNARE proteins (synaptobrevin, syntaxin and SNAP25B) releasing the neurotransmitter acetylcholine to the synaptic cleft (Chen and Scheller 2001). The calcium current persists until the membrane potential is returned to normal by outward fluxes of potassium. Munc18-1 is a chaperone that binds to a self-inhibited "closed" conformation of syntaxin-1B and to SNARE complexes (Lai et al. 2017). Munc13-1, is believed to be involved in synaptic vesicle priming prior to vesicle fusion by catalysing the transition of syntaxin 1B from a closed configuration with Munc18-1 into an open state ready to form SNARE complexes and fuse rapidly. The core SNARE complex, a 4-α helix structure formed by the synaptic vesicle-associated synaptobrevin (v-SNARE) and the presynaptic SNAP25B and syntaxin 1B (t-SNARES) proteins, brings the vesicle and plasma membranes together. Finally, calcium-bound Synaptotagmin (a vesicle Ca^{2+} sensor) binds to the SNARE complex causing vesicle fusion and exocytosis. Adapted from Ma et al. (2013). Mutations in *SYT2* (Whittaker et al. 2015), *VAMP1* (Salpietro et al. 2017), *SNAP25B* (Shen et al. 2014) and *MUNC13-1* cause presynaptic CMS. A colour version of this figure can be seen in the plate section.

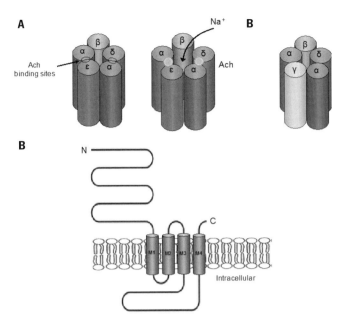

Figure 1.7   Schematic representation of the adult and fetal acetylcholine receptors. A The AChR is made up of five subunits arranged around a central pore. The binding of acetylcholine to the ACh binding sites results in a conformational change that allows the influx of sodium into the muscle and the trigger of an EPP. The fetal AChR has a γ-subunit (green) as opposed to the adult AChR, where the γ-subunit is replaced by an ε-subunit (red). **B** Each AChR subunit is composed of an extracellular domain, four transmembrane domains (M1–M4) and a large cytoplasmic loop that links M3 and M4. ACh, acetylcholine; AChR, acetylcholine receptor; EPP, endplate potential. A colour version of this figure can be seen in the plate section.

acetylcholine binding site located at the α and either δ and ε-subunits interfaces of the AChR (Fig. 7). Upon acetylcholine binding, the AChR subunits undergo a conformational change to open the channel creating a pore (Miyazawa et al. 2003). This event allows the influx of positively charged ions to move across the channel generating a change in the membrane potential that triggers an endplate potential (EPP).

Autoantibodies against the muscle AChR nicotinic receptor cause myasthenia gravis, the most common disorder of neuromuscular transmission (Lindstrom et al. 1976). The AChR antibodies are mostly targeted against the main immunogenic region located in the α-subunit. They cause disease by different pathogenic mechanisms such as complement activation, cross-linking and internalisation of AChRs (Le Panse and Berrih-Aknin 2013). Interestingly, there are patients with autoantibodies against the fetal γ-subunit of the AChR, which is present prenatally but substituted by the ε-subunit before birth, at approximately 33 weeks (AChR γ-to-ε switch) (Missias et al. 1996). As a result, these antibodies have no effect in adults but they can cause neonatal myasthenia (Vernet-Der Garabedian et al. 1994) or arthrogryposis multiplex congenita (Oskoui et al. 2008) via maternal transfer in the fetus.

Mutations in the genes encoding any of the adult AChR subunits can cause AChR deficiency. This is one of the most common congenital myasthenic syndrome (Finlayson 2013), which is characterised by reduced AChR numbers at the endplate (10–30% of normal values) (Vincent et al. 1993). Most of the mutations occur in the ε-subunits and result in protein truncation or loss of essential residues for AChR assembly or function (Abicht et al. 2016). It is believed that incorporation of the fetal AChR γ-subunit into the AChR pentamer enables individuals with null ε-subunits alleles to survive (Cossins et al. 2004). Mutations in the AChR subunits can also alter ion channel function leading to prolonged openings (slow

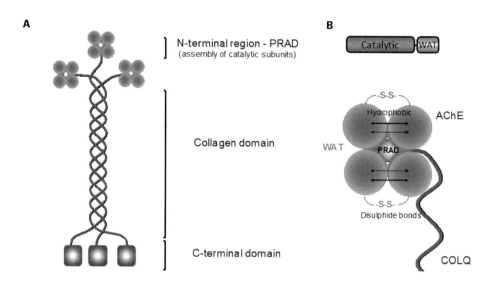

A

N-terminal region - PRAD
(assembly of catalytic subunits)

Collagen domain

C-terminal domain

B

Catalytic WAT

-S-S-
Hydrophobic   AChE

WAT   PRAD

-S-S-
Disulphide bonds

COLQ

Figure 1.8   Schematic representation of acetylcholinesterase and its collagenic-like tail. A ColQ is composed of a N-terminal domain with a Proline Rich Attachment Domain (PRAD) that binds to the catalytic subunits of AChE, a triple-helix collagenic domain, and a C-terminal domain. **B** AChE is composed of a catalytic domain followed by a WAT (tryptophan [W] amphiphilic tetramerisation) domain at the C-terminal region. The association between catalytic subunits is primarily driven by the interaction between WAT domains (green colour) and PRAD (Chen et al. 2011). Additional forces include hydrophobic interactions and disulphide bonds. AChE, acetylcholinesterase. A colour version of this figure can be seen in the plate section.

channel syndrome; SCS) (Ohno et al. 1995) or abbreviated openings (fast channel syndrome; FCS) (Sine et al. 2003).

The Margin of Safety of Neuromuscular Transmission

TThe depolarisation of the postsynaptic membrane that follows the binding of acetylcholine to the AChR generates an endplate potential (EPP), which is greater than the threshold needed to activate the $Na_v1.4$ voltage-gated sodium channels that help trigger an action potential (Engel et al. 2015). Under different stresses or conditions, such as the myasthenic disorders, this margin can be affected leading to abnormal neuromuscular transmission and fatigable muscle weakness (Wood and Slater 2001). Finally, the action potential spreads from the motor endplate to the rest of the muscle sarcolemma generating the contraction of the muscle.

Breakdown of Acetylcholine by Acetylcholinesterase

Acetylcholinesterase (AChE) helps to terminate synaptic transmission by breaking down acetylcholine. AChE is linked to the synaptic basal lamina by a collagenic-like tail, also known as ColQ (Fig. 1.8).

THE N-GLYCOSYLATION PATHWAY OF PROTEINS

The *N*-linked glycosylation pathway is a ubiquitous process in eukaryote cells defined by the sequential attachment of sugar moieties to the lipid dolichol, which is then transferred to an asparagine residue in a protein (Fig. 9). Next generation sequencing has aided the discovery of an unexpected relationship between

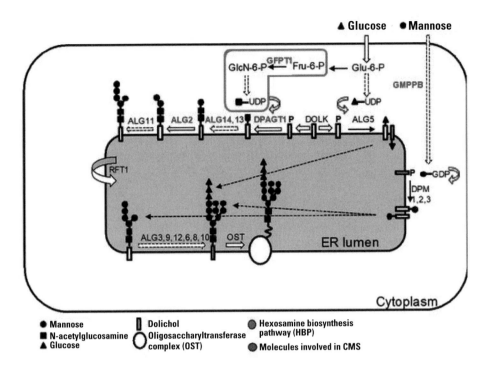

Figure 1.9   Simplified representation of the *N*-glycosylation pathway of proteins. The *N*-linked glycosylation of proteins takes place in the endoplasmic reticulum. It starts with the assembly of the core glycan (*N*-acetylglucosamine, glucose and mannose) on the lipid dolichol. A series of cytosolic glycosyltransferases proceed to dolichol glycosylation on the cytoplasmic face of the endoplasmic reticulum: GFPT1 synthesises UDP-GlcNAc (uridine diphosphate *N*-acetylglucosamine); DPAGT1 and the ALG13/14 complex are involved in adding the first and second *N*-acetylglucosamine to dolichol. Additional sugar residues are added by ALG2 and other enzymes until the resulting product is flipped into the endoplasmic reticulum lumen by RFT1. Inside the endoplasmic reticulum lumen, sugar moieties are incorporated until the glycan is transferred to asparagine residues of nascent proteins by the multimeric oligosaccharyl transferase complex (OST) that subsequently will be modified inside the endoplasmic reticulum and Golgi. DOLK, dolichol kinase; DPM, dolichol-phosphate mannose synthase; Fru-6-P, fructose-6-phosphate; GlcN-6-P, glucosamine-6-phosphate; Glu-6-P, glucose-6-phosphate; GMPPB, GDP-mannose pyrophosphorylase B. Adapted from Rodríguez Cruz (2016) with permission from BMJ Publishing Group Limited. A colour version of this figure can be seen in the plate section.

glycosylation defects in the early stages of the *N*-glycosylation pathway and myasthenic disorders (Senderek et al. 2011; Belaya et al. 2012, 2015). This highlights that genes with no defined function in neuromuscular transmission can also impair the communication between the nerve and the muscle. The reasons why, in certain cases, defects in a ubiquitous process result in dysfunction largely restricted to the NMJ is unclear.

Glycosylation of AChR subunits is required for the correct assembly of AChR pentamers and for efficient export to the cell surface (Gehle et al. 1997) and thus abnormal glycosylation results in reduced AChRs at the muscle endplates, which is most likely the primary mechanisms leading to impaired neuromuscular transmission (Zoltowska et al. 2013). Patients with mutations in the glycosylation genes constitute a distinctive clinical group where muscle weakness is often confined to the limb girdles, and classic myasthenic manifestations – such as ptosis, ophthalmoplegia or facial weakness – are not present (Finlayson et al. 2013; Rodríguez Cruz et al. 2016). Concomitant myopathy is often present, which makes it a progressive condition over time.

REFERENCES

Abicht A, Müller JS, Lochmüller H (2016) *Congenital myasthenic syndromes.* In: Adam MP, Ardinger HH, Pagon RA, et al. (Eds), *Gene Reviews®.* Seattle, WA: University of Washington.

Baker RW, Hughson FM (2016) Chaperoning SNARE assembly and disassembly. *Nat Rev Mol Cell Biol* **17:** 465–479.

Barik A, Lu Y, Sathyamurthy A et al. (2014) LRP4 is critical for neuromuscular junction maintenance. *J Neurosci* **34:** 13892–13905.

Barik A, Li L, Sathyamurthy A, Xiong WC, Mei L (2016) Schwann cells in neuromuscular junction formation and maintenance. *J Neurosci* **36:** 9770–9781.

Bauché S, O'Regan S, Azuma Y et al. (2016) Impaired presynaptic high-affinity choline transporter causes a congenital myasthenic syndrome with episodic apnea. *Am J Hum Genet* **99:** 753–761.

Beeson D, Higuchi O, Palace J et al. (2006) Dok-7 mutations underlie neuromuscular junction synaptopathy. *Science* **313:** 1975–1978.

Belaya K, Finlayson S, Slater CR et al. (2012) Mutations in DPAGT1 cause a limb-girdle congenital myasthenic syndrome with tubular aggregates. *Am J Hum Genet* **91:** 193–201.

Belaya K, Rodríguez Cruz PM, Liu WW et al. (2015) Mutations in GMPPB cause congenital myasthenic syndrome and bridge myasthenic disorders with dystroglycanopathies. *Brain* **138:** 2493–2504.

Chen F, Qian L, Yang ZH et al. (2007) Rapsyn interaction with calpain stabilizes AChR clusters at the neuromuscular junction. *Neuron* **55:** 247–260.

Chen YA, Scheller RH (2001) SNARE-mediated membrane fusion. *Nat Rev Mol Cell Biol* **2:** 98–106.

Chen VP, Luk WK, Chan WK et al. (2011) Molecular assembly and biosynthesis of acetylcholinesterase in brain and muscle: the roles of t-peptide, FHB domain, and N-linked glycosylation. *Front Mol Neurosci* **4:** 36.

Cossins J, Webster R, Maxwell S et al. (2004) A mouse model of AChR deficiency syndrome with a phenotype reflecting the human condition. *Hum Mol Genet* **13:** 2947–2957.

Desaki J, Uehara Y (1981) The overall morphology of neuromuscular junctions as revealed by scanning electron microscopy. *J Neurocytol* **10:** 101–110.

Eaton LM, Lambert EH (1957) Electromyography and electric stimulation of nerves in diseases of motor unit; observations on myasthenic syndrome associated with malignant tumors. *J Am Med Assoc* **163:** 1117–1124.

Engel AG, Shen XM, Selcen D, Sine SM (2015) Congenital myasthenic syndromes: pathogenesis, diagnosis, and treatment. *Lancet Neurol* **14:** 420–434.

Feng Z, Ko C-P (2008) The role of glial cells in the formation and maintenance of the neuromuscular junction. *Ann N Y Acad Sci* **1132:** 19–28.

Finlayson S, Beeson D, Palace J (2013) Congenital myasthenic syndromes: an update. *Pract Neurol* **13:** 80–91.

Finlayson S, Palace J, Belaya K et al. (2013) Clinical features of congenital myasthenic syndrome due to mutations in DPAGT1. *J Neurol Neurosurg Psychiatry* **84:** 1119–1125.

Gehle VM, Walcott EC, Nishizaki T, Sumikawa K (1997) N-glycosylation at the conserved sites ensures the expression of properly folded functional ACh receptors. *Brain Res Mol Brain Res* **45:** 219–229.

De Harven E, Coers C (1959) Electron microscope study of the human neuromuscular junction. *J Biophys Biochem Cytol* **6:** 7–10.

Hoch W, McConville J, Helms S, Newsom-Davis J, Melms A, Vincent A (2001) Auto-antibodies to the receptor tyrosine kinase MuSK in patients with myasthenia gravis without acetylcholine receptor antibodies. *Nat Med* **7:** 365–368.

Jones RA, Harrison C, Eaton SL et al. (2017) Cellular and molecular anatomy of the human neuromuscular junction. *Cell Rep* **21:** 2348–2356.

Karlin A (2002) Emerging structure of the nicotinic acetylcholine receptors. *Nat Rev Neurosci* **3:** 102–114.

Kim N, Stiegler AL, Cameron TO et al. (2008) Lrp4 is a receptor for Agrin and forms a complex with MuSK. *Cell* **135:** 334–342.

Lai Y, Choi UB, Leitz J et al. (2017) Molecular mechanisms of synaptic vesicle priming by Munc13 and Munc18. *Neuron* **95:** 591–607.e10.

Le Panse R, Berrih-Aknin S (2013) Autoimmune myasthenia gravis: autoantibody mechanisms and new developments on immune regulation. *Curr Opin Neurol* **26:** 569–576.

Lin W, Burgess RW, Dominguez B, Pfaff SL, Sanes JR, Lee KF (2001) Distinct roles of nerve and muscle in postsynaptic differentiation of the neuromuscular synapse. *Nature* **410**: 1057–1064.

Lin W, Dominguez B, Yang J et al. (2005) Neurotransmitter acetylcholine negatively regulates neuromuscular synapse formation by a Cdk5-dependent mechanism. *Neuron* **46**: 569–579.

Lindstrom JM, Seybold ME, Lennon VA, Whittingham S, Duane DD (1976) Antibody to acetylcholine receptor in myasthenia gravis. Prevalence, clinical correlates, and diagnostic value. *Neurology* **26**: 1054–1059.

Ma C, Su L, Seven AB, Xu Y, Rizo J (2013) Reconstitution of the vital functions of Munc18 and Munc13 in neurotransmitter release. *Science* **339**: 421–425.

McMahan UJ (1990) The agrin hypothesis. *Cold Spring Harb Symp Quant Biol* **55**: 407–418.

Missias AC, Chu GC, Klocke BJ, Sanes JR, Merlie JP (1996) Maturation of the acetylcholine receptor in skeletal muscle: regulation of the AChR γ-to-∈ switch. *Dev Biol* **179**: 223–238.

Miyazawa A, Fujiyoshi Y, Unwin N (2003) Structure and gating mechanism of the acetylcholine receptor pore. *Nature* **423**: 949–955.

Nachmansohn D, Machado A (1943) The formation of acetylcholine. A new enzyme: "choline acetylase". *J Neurophysiol* **5**: 397–403.

Ohno K, Hutchinson DO, Milone M et al. (1995) Congenital myasthenic syndrome caused by prolonged acetylcholine receptor channel openings due to a mutation in the M2 domain of the ∈ subunit. *Proc Natl Acad Sci USA* **92**: 758–762.

Ohno K, Brengman J, Tsujino A, Engel AG (1998) Human endplate acetylcholinesterase deficiency caused by mutations in the collagen-like tail subunit (ColQ) of the asymmetric enzyme. *Proc Natl Acad Sci USA* **95**: 9654–9659.

Ohno K, Tsujino A, Brengman JM et al. (2001) Choline acetyltransferase mutations cause myasthenic syndrome associated with episodic apnea in humans. *Proc Natl Acad Sci USA* **98**: 2017–2022.

Okada K, Inoue A, Okada M et al. (2006) The muscle protein Dok-7 is essential for neuromuscular synaptogenesis. *Science* **312**: 1802–1805.

Oskoui M, Jacobson L, Chung WK et al. (2008) Fetal acetylcholine receptor inactivation syndrome and maternal myasthenia gravis. *Neurology* **71**: 2010–2012.

Patrick GN, Zukerberg L, Nikolic M, de la Monte S, Dikkes P, Tsai L-H (1999) Conversion of p35 to p25 deregulates Cdk5 activity and promotes neurodegeneration. *Nature* **402**: 615–622.

Rodríguez Cruz PM, Belaya K, Basiri K et al. (2016) Clinical features of the myasthenic syndrome arising from mu- tations in GMPPB. *J Neurol Neurosurg Psychiatry* **87**: 802–809.

Rodríguez Cruz PM, Palace J, Beeson D (2018) The Neuromuscular junction and wide heterogeneity of congenital myasthenic syndromes. *Int. J. Mol.* Sci. **19**: 1677.

Roghani A, Feldman J, Kohan SA et al. (1994) Molecular cloning of a putative vesicular transporter for acetylcholine. *Proc Natl Acad Sci USA* **91**: 10620–10624.

Salpietro V, Lin W, Delle Vedove A et al. (2017) Homozygous mutations in VAMP1 cause a presynaptic congenital myasthenic syndrome. *Ann Neurol* **81**: 597–603.

Sanes JR (2003) The basement membrane/basal lamina of skeletal muscle. *J Biol Chem* **278**: 12601–12604.

Santosa KB, Keane AM, Jablonka-Shariff A, Vannucci B, Snyder-Warwick AK (2018) Clinical relevance of terminal Schwann cells: an overlooked component of the neuromuscular junction. *J Neurosci Res* **96**: 1125–1135.

Senderek J, Müller JS, Dusl M et al. (2011) Hexosamine biosynthetic pathway mutations cause neuromuscular transmission defect. *Am J Hum Genet* **88**: 162–172.

Shen XM, Selcen D, Brengman J, Engel AG (2014) Mutant SNAP25B causes myasthenia, cortical hyperexcitability, ataxia, and intellectual disability. *Neurology* **83**: 2247–2255.

Shi L, Fu AKY, Ip NY (2012) Molecular mechanisms underlying maturation and maintenance of the vertebrate neuromuscular junction. *Trends Neurosci* **35**: 441–453.

Sine SM, Wang HL, Ohno K, Shen XM, Lee WY, Engel AG (2003) Mechanistic diversity underlying fast channel congenital myasthenic syndromes. *Ann N Y Acad Sci* **998**: 128–137.

Slater CR (2017) The structure of human neuromuscular junctions: some unanswered molecular questions. *Int J Mol Sci* **18**: E2183.

Südhof TC (2012) The presynaptic active zone. *Neuron* **75:** 11–25.

Tezuka T, Inoue A, Hoshi T et al. (2014) The MuSK activator agrin has a separate role essential for postnatal mainte-nance of neuromuscular synapses. *Proc Natl Acad Sci USA* **111:** 16556–16561.

Vernet-der Garabedian B, Lacokova M, Eymard B et al. (1994) Association of neonatal myasthenia gravis with antibodies against the fetal acetylcholine receptor. *J Clin Invest* **94:** 555–559.

Vincent A, Newsom-Davis J, Wray D et al. (1993) Clinical and experimental observations in patients with congenital myasthenic syndromes. *Ann N Y Acad Sc* **681:** 451–460.

Whittaker RG, Herrmann DN, Bansagi B et al. (2015) Electrophysiologic features of SYT2 mutations causing a treatable neuromuscular syndrome. *Neurology* **85:** 1964–1971.

Wood SJ, Slater CR (2001) Safety factor at the neuromuscular junction. *Prog Neurobiol* **64:** 393–429.

Wu H, Xiong WC, Mei L (2010) To build a synapse: signaling pathways in neuromuscular junction assembly. *Development* **137:** 1017–1033.

Yang X, Arber S, William C et al. (2001) Patterning of muscle acetylcholine receptor gene expression in the absence of motor innervation. *Neuron* **30:** 399–410.

Zoltowska K, Webster R, Finlayson S et al. (2013) Mutations in GFPT1 that underlie limb-girdle congenital myasthenic syndrome result in reduced cell-surface expression of muscle AChR. *Hum Mol Genet* **22:** 2905–2913.

Zuber B, Unwin N (2013) Structure and superorganization of acetylcholine receptor-rapsyn complexes. *Proc Natl Acad Sci USA* **110:** 10622–10627.

Neurophysiology of Neuromuscular Transmission and its Defects in Children

Matthew Pitt

NORMAL PHYSIOLOGY OF THE NEUROMUSCULAR JUNCTION

The function of the neuromuscular junction (NMJ) is to conduct the effect of the action potential from the nerve to the muscle to produce a similar action potential on the other side. The wave of nerve depolarisation reaches the presynaptic area and here it interacts with calcium and the vesicles containing acetyl choline (ACh) that are stored in that area. These are stimulated to coalesce with the presynaptic membrane releasing ACh into the synaptic cleft. At stimulation rates greater than five per second (see Neurophysiological assessment of neuromuscular transmission section), calcium levels in the presynaptic region do not have sufficient time to return to their baseline values. This results in high calcium concentrations in the presynaptic region, which stimulates release of increased amounts of acetyl choline. This produces the phenomenon of post-tetanic facilitation. The increased demands that this places on the amounts of stored acetyl choline in the presynaptic region mean that this phenomenon is followed by a period of reduced release of acetyl choline and, the so-called, post-tetanic exhaustion.

ACh binds to the receptors on the postsynaptic region causing an endplate potential (EPP). This EPP, if exceeding the threshold for depolarisation of the muscle fibre, will cause an all-or-nothing response. The amount by which the EPP exceeds the threshold is called the safety factor. If the safety factor is exceeded, the EPP will cause a depolarisation of the postsynaptic membrane and generate a muscle action potential (MAP). As this is an-all-or-nothing response, the MAP will have exactly the same amplitude irrespective of the degree by which the safety factor is exceeded.

ACh is released from the receptors after it has affected depolarisation and is acted upon by cholinesterase in the synaptic cleft to be broken down into choline and acetic acid. Choline is reabsorbed into the presynaptic region where it is acted upon by choline acetyl transferase (ChAT) reforming the ACh and replenishing the vesicles ready for the next action potential (Dumitru 1994; Howard 2002; Zwarts 2017) For effective depolarisation of the muscle, the endplates need to be concentrated into a motor unit.

ABNORMAL PHYSIOLOGY OF THE NEUROMUSCULAR JUNCTION

Any part of the process described can be affected leading to a myasthenic condition. Autoimmune myasthenic conditions may be due to anti-acetylcholine receptor(AChR) antibodies or anti-muscle specific kinase (MuSK) antibodies affecting the postsynaptic membrane.

The congenital myasthenic syndromes (CMS) are more variable in their sites of action and any point in the process may be affected by genetic defects which result in abnormalities of the related proteins affecting the structure or function of the AChR (Engel et al. 2015; Beeson 2016; Natera-de Benito et al. 2017; Yiş et al. 2017). Thus, ChAT may be affected causing a failure to produce ACh and a presynaptic dysfunction (Ohno et al. 2001). Deficiency of acetylcholinesterase (Aldunate et al. 2004) in the synaptic cleft may prevent removal of ACh and its breakdown into its component parts of choline and acetic acid causing a hyper-polarisation of the postsynaptic membrane. As with the autoimmune conditions, the bulk of congenital abnormalities affect the postsynaptic region. Some affect the ACh receptor itself with abnormalities of the individual subunits, of which the ε-subunit is most commonly involved (Finlayson et al. 2013). Others affect the means by which the receptors open and close; the so-called fast channel (Sine et al. 2003) and slow channel CMS (Hantai et al. 2004). In addition a significant number of CMS (Lin et al. 2001; Muller et al. 2003, 2006; Nicole et al. 2014; Hurst and Gooch 2016) affect the clustering of the AChR and therefore grouping of the EPPs and the production of a motor unit.

NEUROPHYSIOLOGICAL ASSESSMENT OF NEUROMUSCULAR TRANSMISSION

The electrochemical nature by which a MAP is generated from a descending nerve action potential lends itself to demonstration using neurophysiological techniques. Of the two techniques available, repetitive nerve stimulation (RNS) is the most established (Jolly 1895; Harvey and Masland 1941; Shapiro and Preston 2003) in comparison with single fibre electromyogram (SFEMG), which is a more recent discovery (Stalberg and Ekstedt 1971; Stalberg 1978; Stalberg and Karlsson 2001). The mechanisms by which RNS and SFEMG test the NMJ are similar but subtly different. In RNS the success of the technique depends on abnormalities of the safety factor. This can be best explained by a description of the changes which occur in a normal NMJ (Schumm and Stohr 1984; Schady and MacDermott 1992; Pitt 2017a). In order not to contaminate the changes in the presynaptic region from the effects of calcium uptake, which will enhance the amount of ACh released, the studies for RNS are commenced at a stimulation frequency of 3Hz. This ensures that the abnormalities will reflect only the amount of ACh stored. The calcium concentration in the presynaptic region will be restored to baseline in around 0.2 seconds. Therefore stimulation rates below 5Hz will be unaffected by the enhanced ACh release. The changes in a normal NMJ are demonstrated in Figure 2.1. At 3Hz the release of quanta of ACh follows a pattern. After the initial stimulus, at around the fourth or fifth stimulus, the amount of ACh released in response to individual stimuli reaches a nadir after which a plateau is achieved at a slightly higher level. The EPPs generated in the postsynaptic region, shown in on the left of the illustration, exactly match the amount of ACh released. In the standard RNS protocol, the next manoeuvre is to give tetanic stimulation at rates exceeding 10Hz for a few minutes. This may also be effected by asking the subject to contract the muscle strongly for a short time, which produces a stimulation rate at around 20Hz and is less unpleasant than electrical stimulation. Unfortunately, in children this is not always possible and this then has to be done electrically. Tetanic stimulation will cause an enhanced release of ACh from the increased input of calcium. This means that the potential amplitudes of the EPPs will be increased, the so-called post-tetanic facilitation. In health, because the safety factor is exceeded only by a further degree, this has no effect on the MAP produced, which will be identical. Post-tetanic facilitation is followed by post-tetanic exhaustion with a reduction in the ACh released and a consequent reduction in the EPP. Once again, the degree by which the safety factor is exceeded is irrelevant provided it is exceeded and therefore the MAP in health sees no change during the

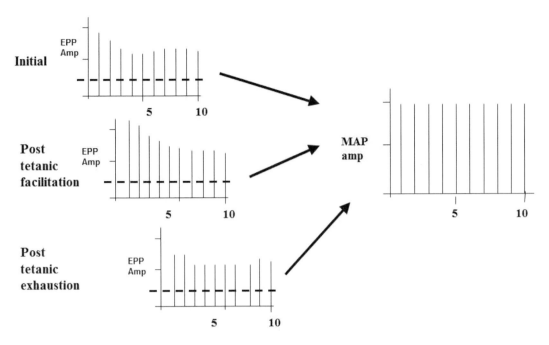

Figure 2.1   Demonstration of the relationship between the amplitude of the endplate potentials (EPPs) and single muscle fibre action potentials (MAPs) following repetitive stimulation at 3Hz. The threshold for depolarisation is shown by the dashed line. Adapted from Figure 9.3 from Pitt (2017a) with permission from Oxford University Press.

three stages of repetitive nerve stimulation: basal rate stimulation, the effect of tetanic stimulation and the period immediately afterwards.

The principle of SFEMG is as follows. When a concentric needle electrode (CNE) is placed into a muscle and the subject contracts that muscle, an interference pattern is produced, which is made up of the motor unit potentials from around the 9 or 10 motor units within range of the CNE. Not all of the muscle fibres within a motor unit will be detected by the needle, which is moved through the muscle in order to recruit different motor units. By either increasing the low-frequency filter or reducing the area of recording surface in the needle it is possible to only recruit action potentials from those fibres nearest the needle. Muscle fibres from an individual motor unit are demonstrated in Figure 2.2. As the action potential propagates down the nerve it reaches the point where it will pass down the two branches, reaching the muscle fibres at slightly different times. Each repetition of this process will produce a MAP in the muscle fibre, whose timing will be slightly different from those that preceded it. The degree of variability as shown here is termed jitter. In Figure 2.2, this particular mechanism is relevant to one single fibre methodology technique called volitional SFEMG. This requires the subject to contract the muscle just sufficiently for the operator to focus on the action potentials and record a steady contraction for sufficient time to measure the jitter. This is very difficult to perform even in adults and is essentially impossible in children under 8 years. Therefore, it does not form the basis of a viable technique for assessment of NMJ disorders in children. Instead we use the technique where the volitional element is removed by stimulating the nerve fibre (Trontelj et al. 1988). The disadvantage is that it is not possible to isolate individual muscle fibres from individual motor units. Instead a response is recorded that is the overlap of MAPs from multiple motor

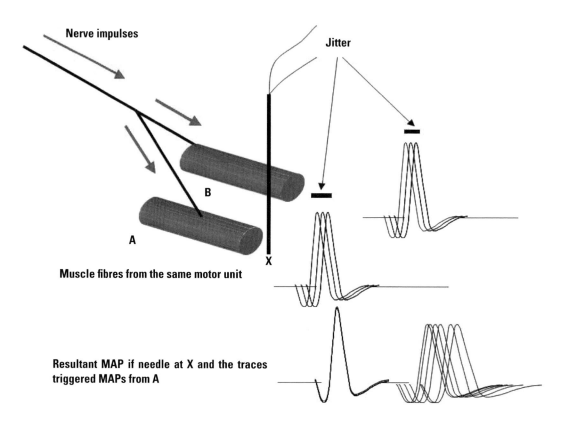

Figure 2.2   Single fibre electromyogram. MAPs from two muscle fibres from the same motor unit showing the variability of the MAP latency with repeated stimulation "jitter". When the recording screen is triggered by the MAP from fibre A, the "jitter" is the summation of two muscle fibres jitter. Adapted from Figure 9.11 from Pitt (2017a) with permission from Oxford University Press.

fibres from several motor units. The technique, however, is eminently practicable and its interpretation allows easy distinction between normality and abnormality in the NMJ.

ELECTROMYOGRAPHY IN MYASTHENIC CONDITIONS

The situation changes completely when the relationship between the EPP and the threshold is altered. In a presynaptic abnormality, the amount of ACh released is reduced while the threshold in the postsynaptic region remains unchanged. If it is likely that the threshold is not reached for depolarisation of the postsynaptic muscle membrane, this is most likely to occur in the basal stimulation at around stimulus four. This will cause a failure of depolarisation of the muscle membrane and, for that particular muscle fibre, the fourth will not be associated with a MAP. In a presynaptic disorder the increase of the ACh released in the response to calcium may overcome this abnormality but afterwards with post-tetanic exhaustion the likelihood that the safety factor is not reached increases. Therefore, in the case of a presynaptic pattern of abnormality, basal studies can be normal or show an abnormality around the fourth stimulus. In a large cohort of adults with Lambert–Eaton syndrome, 99% shown significant decrement at 3Hz (Juel et al. 2006). This is often reversed completely with normalisation, possibly even super-normalisation, of the response when tetanic stimulation is performed only to see the transmission fail with an effect on the MAP generation in the period after tetanic stimulation. What is described here is the effects on individual muscle fibres, but the RNS is recorded from the compound muscle action potential (CMAP) which is the summation of all the muscle action potentials in the muscle in question. Some muscle fibres may be affected more than others but the tendency is that those around the fourth stimuli at 3Hz will to show the most abnormality and therefore a reduction of greater than 10% in that potential, in relation to the initial potential, is considered abnormal. The decline in the amplitude of the CMAP is smooth and gradual, a feature that distinguishes it from the effects of movement, which are random.

In a postsynaptic abnormality, the amount of ACh released is unchanged but the threshold is increased. Once again, the safety factor for the effective transmission of the EEP to the postsynaptic membrane is at risk and those stimuli around the fourth will show this first. In a way analogous to the presynaptic abnormality, basal studies may show a minor change, but this will be effectively corrected by tetanic stimulation only to be worsened in the period immediately afterwards. The distinguishing feature between these two conditions, pre-and postsynaptic abnormalities, is that in the former the CMAP amplitude at the beginning is lower. It may show a dramatic increase with tetanic facilitation up to around 200% of the pre-tetanic level.

One of the most important points about RNS is that it has to be accompanied by failure of transmission across the NMJ for it to be abnormal. This in itself requires a degree of abnormality, which, while often found in many cases of myasthenic weakness, is not seen in every case. It is therefore relatively insensitive (Oh et al. 1992; Lyu et al. 1993; Witoonpanich et al. 2011; Lo et al. 2017) compared with SFEMG, in which the mechanism of detection of an abnormality is different. (Stalberg 1978).

The ways that neuromuscular transmission abnormalities are reflected in changes in the jitter are shown in Figure 2.3. The Figure shows on the left the normal situation where the depolarisations of the muscle membrane and the resulting MAPs produced take place in a relatively short time period. The time it takes for the membrane to reach the threshold for depolarisation is directly proportional to the effective ACh presented to the postsynaptic membrane. In health, this effective concentration varies little and the jitter therefore is relatively small. In NMJ disease, irrespective of whether this is a presynaptic abnormality of ACh release or a postsynaptic abnormality, where the threshold is increased, the effective ACh reaching the postsynaptic membrane varies more than normal and jitter will reflect this by being increased. The most important point, however, is that the transmission of the nerve action potential to the postsynaptic depolarisation of the muscle takes place but it is shown to vary in its timing. For this reason single fibre methodology, which does not require failure of depolarisation of the postsynaptic membrane to be positive, is both theoretically and empirically more likely to be positive than RNS thus making SFEMG a more sensitive diagnostic test than RNS.

PRACTICALITIES OF REPETITIVE NERVE STIMULATION AND SINGLE FIBRE ELECTROMYOGRAPHY IN CHILDREN

RNS is feasible in children although it is very uncomfortable and many practitioners prefer not to use it. The often quoted statement that it will always be positive in a weak muscle is not borne out by either practical experience or the reported sensitivity values in known myasthenics. If decrement can be demonstrated on RNS, however, it is significant, making RNS a highly specific test of neuromuscular transmission defects.

Stimulation SFEMG is the preferred technique to use in children. It is performed on the orbicularis oculi with stimulation of the facial nerve. For reasons of accuracy of nomenclature, it is termed stimulated

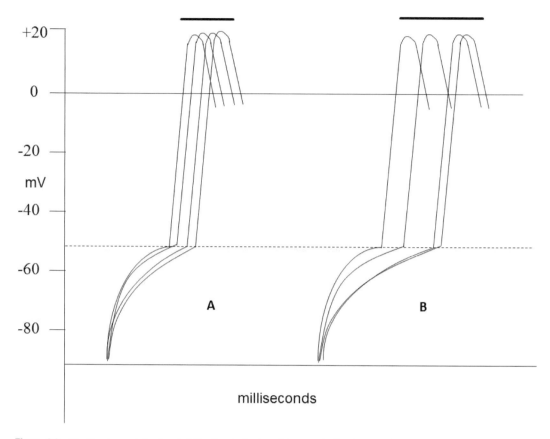

Figure 2.3   The time to reach the threshold for depolarisation of the muscle fibre is proportional to the effective concentration of acetyl choline at the neuromuscular junction. In a normal neuromuscular junction there is little variability **A** in jitter, but in an abnormal neuromuscular junction where the effective concentration is reduced either by reduction in release of acetyl choline (presynaptic abnormality) or an abnormality of the postsynaptic membrane this variability is increased **B**. Adapted from Figure 9.13 from Pitt (2017a) with permission from Oxford University Press.

potential analysis using concentric needle electrodes (SPACE) which is a more accurate description of the technique used (Pitt 2017b; Pitt et al. 2017). With the coalescence of many potentials from different motor units and their component muscle fibres, the possibility of a potential from an individual single fibre being detected is low and becomes even lower the larger the abnormality of jitter. The concentric needle electrode (CNE) is used now because of risks of prions and other diseases being transmitted by reusable needles; an example of which is the purpose built SFEMG needle. The CNE used are of the finest diameter, the so-called facial needle, and using enhanced low-frequency filters it is possible to emulate the recordings made with the SFEMG needle (Farrugia et al. 2009; Stalberg and Sanders 2009; Stalberg 2012; Patel et al. 2016).

The experience of using SPACE is extensive in our laboratory with published reports including over 600 cases, with a personal experience of twice that number. Results show a sensitivity of around 84% and a specificity of 74%. Sensitivity figures are reduced in our published series (Pitt 2017b; Pitt et al. 2017) because of the inclusion of several cases with *GMPPB* mutation; a newly diagnosed form of CMS which has a limb girdle distribution, and most importantly, no reported abnormality of facial musculature (Belaya et al. 2015; Rodríguez Cruz et al. 2016). When figures are looked at in specific subgroups such as

AIMG, and more common types of CMS, such as those due to mutations in the *RAPSN* gene, figures of sensitivity of around 90% or more are achieved.

One of the criticisms levelled at SFEMG methodologies, particularly in children, is the lack of specificity. This has to be acknowledged as SPACE will be affected by any abnormality between the point of stimulation, in our practice, the facial nerve, and the orbicularis oculi. Abnormalities of jitter are present in disease of the motor nerve, which include mitochondrial disorders, motor neurone diseases, such as spinal muscular atrophy or bulbar palsy, and cranial nerve neuropathy or dis-innervation syndromes. At the other end of the axis, abnormalities within the muscle itself may be associated with disorders of the NMJ (Munot et al. 2010; Forrest et al. 2011; Robb et al. 2011; Klein et al. 2013; Illingworth et al. 2014). However, motor nerve abnormalities are detectable by other means, in particular analysis of the interference pattern and nerve conduction studies. Provided the jitter interpretation takes cognizance of the interference pattern analysis and the peripheral nerve studies and does not use results in patients with abnormalities pointing to these disorders, the specificity can be enhanced with little effect on sensitivity. When looking at the levels of jitter abnormality detected, it is noticeable that those caused by myasthenic conditions are often much more marked than those where the abnormality is incidental to NMJ abnormality in a myopathy. Using a value called the Mean Consecutive Difference index (MCD-I) which is computed by dividing the value for the MCD by the upper limit of normal for age, a receiver operating characteristic (ROC) curve showed a value of over 115% as most likely to be caused by a myasthenic condition (Pitt et al. 2017). If it is under that, it is more likely to be a myopathy with a related disorder of neuromuscular transmission. This allows the clinicians receiving our results to guide their investigations appropriately. In the former situation, screening for myasthenia is the first-line of investigation and in the latter a myopathy should be sought by either genetic testing or a muscle biopsy.

SPACE is performed under local anaesthetic, which prevents the need for general anaesthetic. Also as it is a part of a complete examination of the peripheral neuromuscular system, including nerve stimulation and muscle sampling, the whole electrodiagnostic examination can be performed in one appointment. The test is usually effected in less than 15 minutes and most parents are comfortable with it, as are the children.

CONCLUSIONS

Disorders of the NMJ, which include the myasthenic conditions in children, show electrochemical abnormalities which lend themselves to examination by electromyographic techniques. Of the two techniques available, RNS, although more specific, is uncomfortable and less sensitive than SFEMG. The latter is performed using stimulation of the facial nerve using a technique known as SPACE. This technique is well-tolerated and easily performed in trained hands; it has high sensitivity and specificity and is an essential adjunct to clinicians seeking to diagnose these rare but treatable conditions which often have varied clinical presentations.

REFERENCES

Aldunate R, Casar JC, Brandan E, Inestrosa NC (2004) Structural and functional organization of synaptic acetylcholinesterase. *Brain Re Brain Res Rev* **47**: 96–104.

Beeson D (2016) Congenital myasthenic syndromes: recent advances. *Curr Opin Neurol* **29**: 565–571.

Belaya K, Rodríguez Cruz PM, Liu WW et al. (2015) Mutations in GMPPB cause congenital myasthenic syndrome and bridge myasthenic disorders with dystroglycanopathies. *Brain* **138**: 2493–2504.

Dumitru D (1994) *Neuromuscular Junction Disorders. Electrodiagnostic Medicine.* Philadelphia: Hanley and Belfus.

Engel AG, Shen XM, Selcen D, Sine SM (2015) Congenital myasthenic syndromes: pathogenesis, diagnosis, and treatment. *Lancet Neurol* **14:** 461.

Farrugia ME, Weir AI, Cleary M, Cooper S, Metcalfe R, Mallik A (2009) Concentric and single fiber needle electrodes yield comparable jitter results in myasthenia gravis. *Muscle Nerve* **39:** 579–585.

Finlayson S, Beeson D, Palace J (2013) Congenital myasthenic syndromes: an update. *Pract Neurol* **13:** 80–91.

Forrest KM, Al-Sarraj S, Sewry C et al. (2011) Infantile onset myofibrillar myopathy due to recessive CRYAB mutations. *Neuromuscul Disord* **21:** 37–40.

Hantai D, Richard P, Koenig J, Eymard B (2004) Congenital myasthenic syndromes. *Curr Opin Neurol* **17(5):** 539–551.

Harvey AM, Masland RL (1941) A method for the study of neuromuscular transmission in normal subjects. *Bull John Hopkins Hosp* **68:** 81–93.

Howard JF (2002) Neuromuscular transmission. In: Brown WF, Bolton, CF, Aminoff, MJ (Eds), *Neuromuscular Function and Disease. Basic, Clinical and Electrodiagnostic Aspects.* Philadelphia: WB Saunders.

Hurst RL, Gooch CL (2016) Muscle-specific receptor tyrosine kinase (MuSK) myasthenia gravis. *Curr Neurol Neurosci Rep* **16:** 61.

Illingworth MA, Main M, Pitt M et al. (2014) RYR1-related congenital myopathy with fatigable weakness, responding to pyridostigimine. *Neuromuscul Disord* **24:** 707–712.

Jolly F (1895) Uber myasthenia gravis pseudoparalytica. *Berl Klin Wochenschr* **32:** 1–27.

Juel VC, Massey JM, Sanders DB (2006) Lambert Eaton myasthenic syndrome: findings in 97 patients *Muscle Nerve* **34:** 543.

Klein A, Pitt MC, Mchugh JC et al. (2013) DOK7 congenital myasthenic syndrome in childhood: early diagnostic clues in 23 children. *Neuromuscul Disord* **23:** 883–891.

Lin W, Burgess RW, Dominguez B, Pfaff SL, Sanes JR, Lee KF (2001) Distinct roles of nerve and muscle in postsynaptic differentiation of the neuromuscular synapse. *Nature* **410:** 1057–1064.

Lo YL, Najjar RP, Teo KY, Tow SL, Loo JL, Milea D (2017) A reappraisal of diagnostic tests for myasthenia gravis in a large Asian cohort. *J Neurol Sci* **376:** 153–158.

Lyu RK, Cheng SY, Tang LM (1993) Electrodiagnostic studies in myasthenia gravis. *Changgeng Yi Xue Za Zhi* **16:** 164–169.

Muller JS, Mildner G, Muller-Felber W et al. (2003) Rapsyn N88K is a frequent cause of congenital myasthenic syndromes in European patients. *Neurology* **60:** 1805–1810.

Muller JS, Baumeister SK, Schara U et al. (2006) CHRND mutation causes a congenital myasthenic syndrome by impairing co-clustering of the acetylcholine receptor with rapsyn. *Brain* **129:** 2784–2793.

Munot P, Lashley D, Jungbluth H et al. (2010) Congenital fibre type disproportion associated with mutations in the tropomyosin 3 (TPM3) gene mimicking congenital myasthenia. *Neuromuscul Disord* **20:** 796–800.

Natera-de Benito D, Töpf A, Vilchez JJ et al. (2017) Molecular characterization of congenital myasthenic syndromes in Spain. *Neuromuscul Disord* **27:** 1087–1098.

Nicole S, Chaouch A, Torbergsen T et al. (2014) Agrin mutations lead to a congenital myasthenic syndrome with distal muscle weakness and atrophy. *Brain* **137:** 2429–2443.

Oh SJ, Kim DE, Kuruoglu R, Bradley RJ, Dwyer D (1992) Diagnostic sensitivity of the laboratory tests in myasthenia gravis. *Muscle Nerve* **15:** 720–724.

Ohno K, Tsujino A, Brengman JM et al. (2001) Choline acetyltransferase mutations cause myasthenic syndrome associated with episodic apnea in humans. *Proc Natl Acad Sci USA* **98:** 2017–2022.

Patel A, Gosk M, Pitt M (2016) The effect of different low-frequency filters on concentric needle jitter in stimulated orbicularis oculi. *Muscle Nerve* **54:** 317–319.

Pitt MC (2017a) *Paediatric Electromyography*. Oxford: Oxford University Press.

Pitt MC (2017b) Use of stimulated electromyography in the analysis of the neuromuscular junction in children. *Muscle Nerve* **56:** 841–847.

Pitt MC, McHugh JC, Deeb J, Smith RA (2017) Assessing neuromuscular junction stability from stimulated EMG in children. *Clin Neurophysiol* **128:** 290–296.

Robb SA, Sewry CA, Dowling JJ et al. (2011) Impaired neuromuscular transmission and response to acetylcholinesterase inhibitors in centronuclear myopathies. *Neuromuscul Disord* **21:** 379–386.

Rodríguez Cruz PM, Belaya K, Basiri K et al. (2016) Clinical features of the myasthenic syndrome arising from mutations in GMPPB. *J Neurol Neurosurg Psychiatry* **87:** 802–809.

Schady W, MacDermott N (1992) On the choice of muscle in the electrophysiological assessment of myasthenia gravis. *Electromyogr Clin Neurophysiol* **32:** 99–102.

Schumm F, Stohr M (1984) Accessory nerve stimulation in the assessment of myasthenia gravis. *Muscle Nerve* **7:** 147–151.

Shapiro BE, Preston DC (2003) Repetitive nerve stimulation and exercise testing. *Phys Med Rehabil Clin N Am* **14:** 185–206.

Sine SM, Wang HL, Ohno K et al. (2003) Mechanistic diversity underlying fast channel congenital myasthenic syndromes. *Ann N Y Acad Sci* **998:** 128–137.

Stalberg E (1978) Neuromuscular transmission studied with single fibre electromyography. *Acta Anaesthesiol Scand Suppl* **70:** 112–117.

Stalberg E (2012) Jitter analysis with concentric needle electrodes. *Ann N Y Acad Sci* **1274:** 77–85.

Stalberg E, Ekstedt J (1971) Single fibre EMG (clinical experience). *Electroencephalogr Clin Neurophysiol* **30:** 259.

Stalberg E, Karlsson L (2001) Simulation of EMG in pathological situations. *Clin Neurophysiol* **112:** 869–878.

Stalberg EV, Sanders DB (2009) Jitter recordings with concentric needle electrodes. *Muscle Nerve* **40:** 331–339.

Trontelj JV, Khuraibet A, Mihelin M (1988) The jitter in stimulated orbicularis oculi muscle: technique and normal values. *J Neurol Neurosurg Psychiatry* **51:** 814–819.

Witoonpanich R, Dejthevaporn C, Sriphrapradang A, Pulkes T (2011) Electrophysiological and immunological study in myasthenia gravis: diagnostic sensitivity and correlation. *Clin Neurophysiol* **122:** 1873–1877.

Yiş U, Becker K, Kurul SH et al. (2017) Genetic landscape of congenital myasthenic syndromes from Turkey: novel mutations and clinical insights. *J Child Neurol* **32:** 759–765.

Zwarts MJ (2017) Nerve, muscle, and neuromuscular junction. In Mills KR (Ed.) *Oxford Textbook of Clinical Neurophysiology*. Glasgow: Oxford University Press.

Disorders of Neuromuscular Transmission: An Overview

Vamshi K Rao, Nancy L Kuntz

Disorders of neuromuscular transmission, with both genetic and acquired autoimmune and infective aetiologies, occur in infants and children of all ages from birth to adolescence.

INTRODUCTION

Congenital myasthenic syndromes (CMS) are due to genetic mutations with most forms being inherited in an autosomal recessive pattern except for slow channel syndrome, SNAP-25 and synaptotagmin-2 deficiencies which are inherited in a dominant manner (Engel 2018). There is an increased incidence of acquired autoimmune myasthenia gravis in individuals with affected first degree relatives (adjusted relative risk of 7.78 in a Taiwanese study) (Liu et al. 2017). Further, concordance of acquired myasthenia gravis in monozygotic twins was documented to be 35.5% as compared to 4–5% in dizygotic pairs (Ramanujam et al. 2011). All forms of myasthenia are relatively infrequent in children, with estimates of the incidence of myasthenia gravis occurring in children quoted as between 1 and 5 cases per million person years with a higher prevalence in children of Asian as compared to Caucasian ethnicity (Parr et al. 2014; Peragallo 2017). While "myasthenia" refers to fatigable weakness in patients of all ages, the symptom presentation, or its interpretation, can be quite different in children as compared to adults. For example, fatigable ptosis (particularly if symmetric) can be difficult to differentiate from the lowering of eyelids observed in sleepy infants ready to nap. Fatigable muscle weakness needs to be distinguished from tiredness. Isolated fatigable ophthalmoparesis due to myasthenia gravis looks much like the decompensation that occurs in idiopathic strabismus when children are overtired. Fatigable lower extremity weakness caused by myasthenia gravis can be difficult to differentiate from those toddlers who will fall more frequently, refuse to walk or demand to be carried when tired.

Fatigue can be difficult to assess in adolescents who frequently have inadequate hours of sleep, not infrequently skip breakfast and who are frequently overcommitted in terms of academic, social and extra-curricular demands on their lives. In summary, care is needed to differentiate between tiredness or sleepiness on the one hand and postexercise weakness in various muscle groups, which repairs with rest on the other.

TRANSIENT NEONATAL MYASTHENIA GRAVIS

A minority (5–30%) of infants born to mothers with acquired autoimmune myasthenia gravis will have transient neonatal symptoms consisting of variable severity of hypotonia, feeding difficulties and respiratory weakness (Peragallo 2017). Pregnant women with localised (ocular) myasthenia gravis and those without detectable acetylcholine receptor (AchR) or muscle-specific kinase (MuSK) antibodies also have the potential to have transient neonatal myasthenia gravis occur in their newborn infants (Townsel et al. 2016). While a United Kingdom multispecialty task force has recommended observation of neonates at risk for transient neonatal myasthenia gravis for 48 hours (Norwood et al. 2014), a case report of an infant born to a mother in clinical remission with double seronegative ocular myasthenia gravis describes symptoms which presented at 3 days of age (Townsel et al. 2016). Symptoms will respond to treatment with acetylcholinesterase inhibitors or plasma exchange and resolve within several weeks to several months. A recent report described the use of sugammadex in reversing neuromuscular blockade in a 3-week-old boy with pyloric stenosis who underwent pyloromyotomy using rocuronium for neuromuscular blockade during surgery (Rubin and Ramamurthi 2017). Sugammadex, which is not yet available for use in the United States, binds directly with rocuronium.

BOTULISM: FOODBORNE, WOUND AND INFANTILE

Botulinum neurotoxin is extremely potent and the median interval between onset and peak of symptoms is 1–3 days, depending on the type of exposure (Halpin et al. 2017; Griese et al. 2017). The toxin binds irreversibly to one of the SNARE proteins in the presynaptic terminal (depending on the specific subtype), preventing acetylcholine release and causing failure of neuromuscular transmission (Rosow and Strober 2015). While foodborne and wound botulism occur with the same pathophysiology as in adults, infantile botulism is unique and occurs when infants ingest botulinum spores which produce and release toxin in the infant's intestine. Although all subtypes have been reported to cause illness in children, the most common are types A and B. Type F has been reported to cause a clinically significant but relatively small proportion of infantile botulism cases, characterised by very young age, rapid progression and severe weakness (Halpin et al. 2017). Symptoms of botulism consist of bilateral cranial nerve palsies, dysphagia, hypotonia, respiratory weakness and flaccid paralysis. Symptoms, such as diplopia or dry mouth, which can differentiate infantile botulism from other clinical mimics, such as spinal muscular atrophy or certain metabolic disorders (Khouri et al. 2018), will not be freely reported by infants and young children. Mortality has gradually declined from 23% (reported in a review of experience from 1929 to 2015) to less than 1% in the most prevalent form (infantile botulism) in the United States in recent years (Rosow and Strober 2015; Griese et al. 2017). Improvement in prognosis has occurred as a result of prompt clinical recognition, provision of needed intensive care and availability of antitoxin. A major challenge to prompt diagnosis has been the time required to perform the toxin neutralisation bioassay in mice (up to 10 days) or to obtain polymerase chain reaction (PCR) or enzyme-linked immunosorbent assay (ELISA) confirmation of the toxin (up to 3 days). Neurophysiological testing can be helpful in confirming a presynaptic defect in neuromuscular transmission without waiting for confirmatory biologic testing (Cornblath et al. 1983). Gutierrez and colleagues characterised the profile in infantile botulism: low amplitude compound muscle action potential (CMAP) in association with tetanic facilitation of amplitude (at least 20% increase) with a duration of post-tetanic facilitation lasting at least 2 minutes (Gutierrez et al. 1994). Verma and colleagues have demonstrated blocking and increased mean jitter with stimulated jitter analysis (assessment of jitter using single fiber emyasthenia gravis filter settings with a concentric needle recording electrode) in small numbers of infants with botulism (Verma and Lin 2016). Although the majority of the published literature relates to cases in the United States, botulism has been reported in infants and children from at least 35 countries (all continents except for Africa and Antarctica) (Drivenes et al. 2017; Griese et al. 2017). Treatment with antitoxin has led to significant improvement in outcomes as it binds to circulating toxin and prevents additional damage to the presynaptic terminal while the process of gradual repair begins (Rosow and Strober 2015).

JUVENILE MYASTHENIA GRAVIS

Children with generalised myasthenia gravis (frequently referred to as having juvenile myasthenia gravis or JMG) can have detectable serum antibodies against components of the AchR, MuSK, lipoprotein receptor-related membrane protein 4 (LRP-4) or be seronegative (Peragallo 2017). Generalised myasthenia gravis will be considered in greater detail in subsequent chapters.

OCULAR MYASTHENIA GRAVIS

In children, ocular symptoms are frequently the initial clinical symptom of myasthenia gravis. Ocular myasthenia gravis (OMG) occurs significantly more frequently in children of Asian ethnicity than other ethnicities. About 50% of these children progress to demonstrating generalised myasthenia gravis within 2 years (Evoli et al. 2017). However, the subset of children with ocular involvement from MuSK-antibody associated myasthenia gravis overwhelmingly progress to have generalised weakness (Skjei et al. 2013). Musk-antibody associated myasthenia gravis typically causes bilateral and symmetric ophthalmoparesis (Evoli et al. 2017).

Children with ophthalmoparesis, or severe ptosis as symptoms of myasthenia gravis, need to be carefully monitored by ophthalmology in order to prevent the development of amblyopia.

LAMBERT–EATON MYASTHENIC SYNDROME

Lambert–Eaton myasthenic syndrome (LEMS) is a condition in which muscle weakness and autonomic symptoms occur due to defective presynaptic release of acetylcholine. Antibodies against the P/Q type voltage-gated calcium channel are detected in the majority of affected individuals. LEMS usually presents in adults as a paraneoplastic syndrome (with small cell lung cancer frequently underlying the clinical symptoms). A handful of children have been described with an underlying neuroblastoma but this is a small fraction of the total cases of LEMS described in children, most of who have other autoimmune conditions in addition to LEMS (Morgan-Followell and de Los Reyes 2013; Verbeek et al. 2014). The key to diagnosis of LEMS lies with the clear improvement of muscle strength, muscle stretch reflexes and CMAP amplitudes in response to brief intervals of exercise. A recent review confirmed the neurophysiologic profile in LEMS which includes low CMAP amplitudes, increment in amplitude (≥60%) with high rates of repetitive stimulation or exercise and decrement in amplitude with low-rate stimulation (Oh 2017).

CONGENITAL MYASTHENIC SYNDROMES

Congenital myasthenic syndromes (CMS) are anatomic or physiologic deficiencies in the neuromuscular transmission apparatus caused by single gene defects (Engel 2018). While each of the individual types is rare, over 25 different causative genes have been identified (Lee et al. 2018). Cumulative prevalence of all types of CMS in children in the United Kingdom has been estimated to be 9.2 cases per million (Parr et al. 2014). Slow channel syndrome and deficiencies of SNAP25 and synaptotagmin-2 are inherited as an autosomal dominant disorder with all other described forms of CMS being inherited as recessive conditions. Each of these genetic defects are present from birth with neonatal onset symptoms of hypotonia, weakness (particularly bulbar and respiratory) and ophthalmoparesis. Some types of CMS present later in infancy (choline acetyltransferase deficiency causing apnoea after crying) or in the childhood to adult years (SCN4A causing episodes of weakness; DOK-7 or agrin deficiencies causing a limb-girdle weakness)

(Souza et al. 2016). As will be described in more detail in later chapters, a number of forms of CMS respond to pharmacologic treatments; however, care is required as medications which are therapeutic in some forms of CMS can cause clinical worsening in others (Lee et al. 2018).

MYOPATHIES WITH SECONDARY NEUROMUSCULAR TRANSMISSION DEFECTS

It has recently been recognised that some forms of congenital myopathy, congenital muscular dystrophies or congenital disorders of glycosylation have a physiologic defects in neuromuscular transmission which cause clinical fatigability and respond to pharmacologic treatment similar to myasthenia (Souza et al. 2016). These will be described in greater detail in a later chapter.

TREATMENT AND ANTICIPATORY GUIDANCE

School-aged children and adolescents will sometimes deny or mask their symptoms in order to avoid drawing attention to the fact that they function differently from their peers. Younger children think concretely and can worry that some minor behavioural infraction or bad thought has caused a newly emerging symptom. These behavioural tendencies create a potential barrier to early identification and treatment of myasthenic conditions. In addition, a poorly coordinated, stumbling young adult with droopy eyes and slurred speech can easily be assumed to be intoxicated rather than potentially having myasthenia. Parents can worry about "crying wolf" or activating the emergency medical system too early only to recognise that their child is not truly in crisis. All of these issues need to be discussed frankly between parents, their child with myasthenia gravis and the treating medical specialist in order to ensure that early evaluation will always be sought with new or changing symptoms.

Symptomatic treatment includes assuring adequate rest periods, spacing of physically vigorous activities and providing any needed nutritional or respiratory support measures to children with any form of myasthenia. Development of emergency action plans (for school and in the community), including discussions with emergency medical service providers, is appropriate. Home and school environments may need individualised spatial adaptations. Pharmacologically, therapy with medications which inhibit acetylcholinesterase function, such as oral pyridostigmine, is beneficial in most infants and children with transient neonatal myasthenia gravis, OMG or generalised myasthenia gravis. On an individualised basis with attention to the specific type of CMS, medications including pyridostigmine, 3,4-diaminopyridine, albuterol (salbutamol), ephedrine, fluoxetine and quinidine are therapeutic.

Immunomodulatory therapies and thymectomy are appropriately limited to autoimmune forms of myasthenia gravis. Plasma exchange and infusions of intravenous immunoglobulin (IVIG) are interventions appropriate for managing myasthenic crises in addition to supportive intensive medical management. In children, where there are additional concerns about the potential of long-term immunosuppressive therapy affecting growth and fertility, plasma exchange (PLEX) and IVIG sometimes play a role in chronic management of autoimmune myasthenia gravis (Sanders et al. 2018). Immuno suppression using oral corticosteroids, azathioprine, mycophenolate and tacrolimus plays a primary therapeutic role for children with autoimmune myasthenia gravis, with frequency of use varying in different parts of the world. Rituximab has been used in refractory autoimmune myasthenia gravis in children although there have been no randomised controlled trials. Treatment of autoimmune myasthenia gravis and CMS in children will be considered in more detail in later chapters.

A meta-analysis of patients with OMG, without underlying thymomas, treated with thymectomy demonstrated an improved rate of complete spontaneous disease remission, speedier recovery and a lower rate of complications in children as compared to adults (Zhu et al. 2017). However, thymectomy is more frequently performed in children with generalised myasthenia gravis. In contrast to adult myasthenia gravis, presence of a thymoma underlying JMG has been described only in rare case reports (Nikolic et al. 2012; Castro et al. 2013). Therefore, in children with autoimmune myasthenia gravis, thymectomy is performed more for the potential to increase long-term rates of clinical remission.

REFERENCES

Castro D, Derisavifard S, Anderson M, Greene M, Iannaccone S (2013) Juvenile myasthenia gravis: a twenty-year experience. *J Clin Neuromuscul Dis* **14:** 95–102.

Cornblath DR, Sladky JT, Sumner AJ (1983) Clinical electrophysiology of infantile botulism. *Muscle Nerve* **6:** 448–452.

Drivenes B, Krause TG, Andersson M et al. (2017) Infant botulism in Denmark from 1995 to 2015. *Dan Med J* **64:** 64.

Engel AG (2018) Genetic basis and phenotypic features of congenital myasthenic syndromes. *Handb Clin Neurol* **148:** 565–589.

Evoli A, Alboini PE, Iorio R, Damato V, Bartoccioni E (2017) Pattern of ocular involvement in myasthenia gravis with MuSK antibodies. *J Neurol Neurosurg Psychiatry* **88:** 761–763.

Griese SE, Kisselburgh HM, Bartenfeld MT et al. (2017) Pediatric botulism and use of equine botulinum antitoxin in children: A systematic review. *Clin Infect Dis* **66(suppl-1):** S17–S29.

Gutierrez AR, Bodensteiner J, Gutmann L (1994) Electrodiagnosis of infantile botulism. *J Child Neurol* **9:** 362–365.

Halpin AL, Khouri JM, Payne JR et al. (2017) Type F infant botulism: investigation of recent clusters and overview of this exceedingly rare disease. *Clin Infect Dis* **66(suppl-1):** S92–S94.

Khouri JM, Payne JR, Arnon SS (2018) More clinical mimics of infant botulism. *J Pediatr* **193:** 178–182.

Lee M, Beeson D, Palace J (2018) Therapeutic strategies for congenital myasthenic syndromes. *Ann N Y Acad Sci* **1412:** 129–136.

Liu FC, Kuo CF, See LC, Tsai HI, Yu HP (2017) Familial aggregation of myasthenia gravis in affected families: a population-based study. *Clin Epidemiol* **9:** 527–535.

Morgan-Followell B, de Los Reyes E (2013) Child neurology: diagnosis of Lambert–Eaton myasthenic syndrome in children. *Neurology* **80:** e220–e222.

Nikolic DM, Nikolic AV, Lavrnic DV, Medjo BP, Ivanovski PI (2012) Childhood-onset myasthenia gravis with thymoma. *Pediatr Neurol* **46:** 329–331.

Norwood F, Dhanjal M, Hill M et al. (2014) Myasthenia in pregnancy: best practice guidelines from a UK multispecialty working group. *J Neurol Neurosurg Psychiatry* **85:** 538–543.

Oh SJ (2017) Distinguishing features of the repetitive nerve stimulation test between Lambert–Eaton myasthenic syndrome and myasthenia gravis, 50-year reappraisal. *J Clin Neuromuscul Dis* **19:** 66–75.

Parr JR, Andrew MJ, Finnis M, Beeson D, Vincent A, Jayawant S (2014) How common is childhood myasthenia? The UK incidence and prevalence of autoimmune and congenital myasthenia. *Arch Dis Child* **99:** 539–542.

Peragallo JH (2017) Pediatric myasthenia gravis. *Semin Pediatr Neurol* **24:** 116–121.

Ramanujam R, Pirskanen R, Ramanujam S, Hammarström L (2011) Utilizing twins concordance rates to infer the predisposition to myasthenia gravis. *Twin Res Hum Genet* **14:** 129–136.

Rosow LK, Strober JB (2015) Infant botulism: review and clinical update. *Pediatr Neurol* **52:** 487–492.

Rubin JE, Ramamurthi RJ (2017) The role of sugammadex in symptomatic transient neonatal myasthenia gravis: a case report. *A Case Rep* **9:** 271–273.

Sanders DB, Wolfe GI, Narayanaswami P (2018) MGFA Task Force on MG Treatment Guidance. Developing treatment guidelines for myasthenia gravis. *Ann N Y Acad Sci* **1412:** 95–101.

Skjei KL, Lennon VA, Kuntz NL (2013) Muscle specific kinase autoimmune myasthenia gravis in children: a case series. *Neuromuscul Disord* **23:** 874–882.

Souza PV, Batistella GN, Lino VC, Pinto WB, Annes M, Oliveira AS (2016) Clinical and genetic basis of congenital myasthenic syndromes. *Arq Neuropsiquiatr* **74:** 750–760.

Townsel C, Keller R, Johnson K, Hussain N, Campbell WA (2016) Seronegative maternal ocular myasthenia gravis and delayed transient neonatal myasthenia gravis. *AJP Rep* **6:** e133–e136.

Verbeek S, Vanakker O, Mercelis R et al. (2014) Lambert–Eaton myasthenic syndrome in a 13-year-old girl with Xp11.22-p11.23 duplication. *Eur J Paediatr Neurol* **18:** 439–443.

Verma S, Lin J (2016) Stimulated jitter analysis for the evaluation of neuromuscular junction disorders in children. *Muscle Nerve* **53:** 471–472.

Zhu K, Li J, Huang X et al. (2017) Thymectomy is a beneficial therapy for patients with non-thymomatous ocular myasthenia gravis: a systematic review and meta-analysis. *Neurol Sci* **38:** 1753–1760.

Epidemiology of Myasthenia in Childhood

Samyami Chowdhury, Jeremy Parr and Sandeep Jayawant

INTRODUCTION AND SUBTYPES

The epidemiology of childhood myasthenia has become much more clearly delineated in the last decade. Historically, much of our knowledge about the incidence and prevalence of myasthenia has been based on studies of adults. However, recent childhood studies from across the world have shown similarities and differences in epidemiology – in part due to methodological differences, but possibly due to genetic and environmental variation between settings (Parr et al. 2014).

Childhood myasthenia includes both autoimmune myasthenia and the congenital myasthenic syndromes. Types of autoimmune myasthenia include neonatal transient myasthenia, juvenile (considered from the first year of life and further divided into prepubertal, pubertal and postpubertal). The disease is caused by the action of autoantibodies on the acetylcholine receptor (AChRs) at the neuromuscular junction (NMJ) causing transmission difficulties. This deficiency in AChRs is the result of an antibody-mediated autoimmune attack. Seropositive refers to the presence of detectable autoantibodies to the acetylcholine receptor AChR or to muscle specific tyrosine kinase protein "MuSK", the latter accounting for approximately 6% of autoimmune myasthenia cases (Zisimopoulou et al. 2014). There is a difference in pathophysiology regarding antibody mediation between AChR and MuSK. Autoantibodies to AChR are thought to activate complement from the IgG1 and IgG3 subclasses of immunoglobulins, whereas the IgG4 subclass is activated in anti-MuSK myasthenia. In adults, MuSK myasthenia has a female preponderance often in the fortieth decade with ocular and or bulbar symptoms present at onset (Weatherbee et al. 2006). A third rare type, is that of double-seronegative myasthenia gravis (dSN-myasthenia gravis) whereby autoantibodies against the low-density lipoprotein receptor-related protein 4 (LRP4) have been identified (Zisimopoulou et al. 2014). This single-pass transmembrane protein has vital roles in development and physiology including neuromuscular synapses, signal transduction and receptor-mediated endocytosis.

Congenital myasthenic syndromes (CMS) are a part of childhood myasthenia. CMS is due to genetic defects encoding proteins that are essential for maintaining the integrity of neuromuscular transmission. There is disrupted signalling between cells resulting in an impaired ability to move skeletal muscles, muscle weakness and delayed development of motor skills (Parr et al. 2014). The most commonly occurring CMS subtypes included those due to mutations in CHRNE, RAPSN and DOK7.

INTERNATIONAL EVIDENCE ABOUT INCIDENCE AND PREVALENCE

Most epidemiological studies published are for the adult population with some children included in them. There are very few published studies in the paediatric population for either congenital or autoimmune myasthenia. We highlight some published studies which are largely adult population-based studies.

United Kingdom

A systematic review of population-based studies of adults and children was conducted by Carr et al. in 2010. This revealed incidence rates of autoimmune myasthenia of 1.7–21.3 per million person-years and prevalence rates of 15–179 per million (Table 4.1). In a study by Parr et al. (2014), the mean incidence of antibody-positive autoimmune myasthenia was 1.5 per million children per year. This study also detected that the prevalence of genetically confirmed CMS was 9.2 per million children under the age of 18. There was no sex difference for CMS. The prevalence of CMS varied across geographical regions in the United Kingdom (between 2.8–14.8 per million children). Regarding autoimmune myasthenic, the mean incidence of antibody-positive autoimmune myasthenia was 1.5 per million children over the period of a study that took place between 2003–2007 (Parr et al. 2014). Much less information is available about the epidemiology of seronegative myasthenia.

Studies in the United Kingdom show no evidence of increasing incidence of autoimmune myasthenia in children (Parr et al. 2014). Girls are more likely than boys to have autoimmune myasthenia both in younger and older age groups. This contrasts with a Turkish study that showed that female sex bias was only present in the older children and with onset after 10 years old.

The prevalence of myasthenia gravis in adults in the United Kingdom is estimated at 15 per 100 000 population with the figures increasing over time. There is a bimodal incidence with female preponderance in the younger adults and male preponderance in the older adults.

Europe

A large Norwegian study investigated the incidence and prevalence of autoimmune myasthenia gravis among children in Norway (Popperud et al. 2017). Popperud and colleagues undertook a retrospective population-based study in Norway from January 2012 to December 2013. Cases of juvenile myasthenia gravis (JMG) with onset less than 18 years were identified through electronic patient records at the 15 main hospitals in Norway between 1989 and 2013. In total 63 unique JMG cases were identified giving an average annual incidence rate of 1.6 per million. The incidence rate was stable over the study period. The prevalence of JMG was 3.6–13.8 per million. The majority of JMG cases were in females. The risk of JMG was higher among females both in the postpubertal and prepubertal groups (Popperud et al. 2017).

In Northern Portugal, the estimated point prevalence of autoimmune myasthenia was 111.7 patients per million population. The incidence rate among men was estimated at 6.3 per million per year. Among women, the incidence rate was highest in 15–49-year-old age group whereas in men the incidence increased with age to 22.1 per million in men aged over 65 years.

Data from Northern Italy with a small sample of 49 patients showed a mean incidence per year of 7.8 per million between 1980 and 1994. The average age at onset was 44.5 ± 21 years and the average age at the time of prevalence determination was 51.1 ± 19.6 years for active disease. The point prevalence rate in 1994 was 117.5 per million for all patients with either active or quiescent disease and 103.4 per million for active disease alone (Ferrari and Lovaste 1992). Ferrari et al. carried out their prevalence study in a geographical area with a population of 444 879; the crude prevalence rate was 7.4 per million per year; 10.8 for females and 4.6 for males. They also found that myasthenia gravis has a female preponderance

Table 4.1 Myasthenia incidence and prevalence table

Country of study (participant age in years)	Incidence (per million/year)	Prevalence (per million)	Adult or paediatric	Reference
United Kingdom	1.5	9.2	Pacdiatric	Parr et al. 2014
Norway	1.6	3.6–13.8	Paediatric	Popperud et al. 2017
Denmark				
0–9	0.3		Adult	Pedersen et al. 2013
10–19	2.2			
Italy				
Bologna & Ferrera				
0–9		17.4	Adult	Casetta et al. 2004
10–19				
Emilia Romagna				
0–14	1.6			Emilia-Romagna study
15–24	5.5			group
Reggio				
0–9	4			Guidetti et al. 1998
10–19	4			
Trento				
0–9	2.1			Ferrari and Lovaste 1992
10–19	1.5			
Sardinia				
0–10	0.2			Aiello et al. 1997
11–20	2.8			
Estonia				
0–9	1		Adult	Oöpik et al. 2003
10–19	4.2			
Yugoslavia				
0–19	0		Adult	Lavrnić et al. 1999
10–19	4.5			
Greece				
0–9		4.71	Adult	Poulas et al. 2001
10–19		14.87		
Sweden[a] (per 100 000)				
0–14		0.3	Adult	Kalb et al. 2002
14–24		4		
Tanzania				
0–19	2.2		Adult	Matuja et al. 2001
Libya				
0–20	3.3		Adult	Radhakrishnan et al. 1988
South Africa	4.3		Adult	Mombaur et al. 2015
China	4	62.2	Adult	Yu et al. 1992
Taiwan				
0–4	0.89	14	Adult	Lai and Tseng 2010
5–9	0.69			
10–14	0.37			
15–19	0.83			
Canada	0.9 (in 2011)	32 (per 100 000)		Breiner et al. 2016
USA		20 (per 100 000)		Phillips 2003

[a]3.7–8.9 in juvenile myasthenia gravis.

with a peak onset at 20–29 years. In Sardinia, the rate of autoimmune myasthenia was 45 per million population in a study of the entire 270 000 Sardinian population by Aiello et al. (1997); the prevalence was 111 per million population: 124 per million in women and 9.9 per million in men. The reported prevalence of myasthenia gravis in Sardinia was higher than shown in previous studies (Aiello et al. 1997).

From 1985 to 2000, Casetta et al. (2004) completed a study in the province of Ferrara, Italy, with a mean population base of 360 950 people. The average crude annual incidence rate of myasthenia gravis was 2 per 100 000 again confirming a female preponderance, particularly in the youngest age groups. Only one case of myasthenia gravis was identified in the 0–14 age group (population 34 672); overall the incidence in this age group was 0.2 per 100 000 (0.4 per 100 000 in women). A prevalence rate of 105.4 cases of myasthenia gravis per million population was reported.

In Denmark, Christensen et al. (1993) investigated a population of 2.8 million and showed an average incidence rate of 5 per million population (women 5.9 and men 4.2). The incidence of myasthenia gravis increased after the age of 40 years. In women, the incidence rate showed a bimodal pattern with a peak of 7 per million in women of age 20–29 years and a second peak of 11.7 per million in those aged 70–79 years. The incidence rates suggest that younger women are more susceptible to myasthenia gravis than younger men (a consistent finding among most epidemiological studies of myasthenia gravis). No data incidence or prevalence data were available for the paediatric population alone.

United States and Canada

In the United States, myasthenia gravis affects 2–10 per 100 000. Before age 40 years, myasthenia gravis is three times more common in women than men. Myasthenia gravis is rare before the age of 10 years, or after 60 years. Once again, a bimodal distribution in incidence was found, with an earlier peak involving women between the ages of 10 and 40 years and men between the ages of 50 and 70 (Jacobson et al. 1997).

In the prepubertal phase, the male:female ratio was equal in patients of northern European descent. It was also reported that the disease in this group is of lesser severity, shorter disease duration and with a higher remission rate; 32% of prepubertal children were found to be seronegative. Postpuberty myasthenia gravis becomes more prevalent in females; the symptomatology was found to be similar to that of adults. The female male ratio is 4.5:1 with females suffering more severe disease compared to men.

Myasthenia gravis is more common in female African–American children of all ages.

The largest population-based epidemiological study of myasthenia gravis in a North American setting was undertaken in Canada by Breiner et al. (2016). They examined the incidence and prevalence of myasthenia gravis across Ontario. The age range did not include any persons less than 18 years old and therefore no data on paediatric myasthenia gravis was given. The study shows rising myasthenia gravis prevalence with stable incidence over time in the adult population. The crude prevalence rate was 32.0 per 100 000 population in 2013. Age- and sex-standardised prevalence rates rose consistently over time from 16.3 per 100 000 (confidence interval 15.4–17.1) in 1996 to 26.3 per 100 000 (confidence interval 25.4–27.3) in 2013 (Breiner et al. 2016).

China and Taiwan

Wang et al. (2013) undertook a cohort study in Beijing over 3 years with 1108 patients with myasthenia gravis (555 males and 553 females). The diversity of clinical features of Chinese patients with myasthenia was related to gene polymorphism of Chinese in the north and south of China: 13.5% of cases were of childhood myasthenia (less than 5 years old); 27.3% of people with myasthenia gravis first presented prior to age 15 years; 62.5% presented as adolescents. Both males and females had a peak incidence before age 5 years; males had a second incidence peak at age 40 years.

Yu et al. (1992) conducted a territory-wide study of myasthenia gravis in Hong Kong, identifying 262 Chinese patients (103 paediatric onset; 159 adult onset). This corresponded to a point prevalence and period prevalence of 53.5 and 62.2 per million respectively with an average annual incidence of 4.0 per million population. There was a female predominance in the whole group of patients (female to male ratio 1.6:1) and in those with adult disease (ratio 2.1:1), but not in those with onset in childhood. Onset of disease was most common in the first three decades of life and became less common in subsequent decades. Nine patients died during the study, seven from myasthenia gravis, giving a case fatality rate of 0.027 per million. (Yu et al. 1997).

Juvenile onset myasthenia gravis occurred in 39.3% of patients and restricted ocular myasthenia gravis in 47.9%. The highest incidence for both sexes was in before age 10 years. In adults, a relatively stable incidence was found, with a slight decline in the fourth decade. There was no significant female predominance in paediatric patients. The evenly balanced sex ratio in paediatric patients was similar to that seen in Taiwan Chinese (Chiu et al. 1987). Importantly, the predominance of disease onset in early life resembles Taiwan Chinese and Japanese but differs from Caucasians. The contrast between Chinese and Caucasian patients was even more marked when disease type was considered. The high prevalence of ocular disease (47.3%), particularly in juvenile patients (71%), was similar to that reported in Taiwan Chinese (Chiu et al. 1987). A lot of data that has been gathered is pre-LRP4 era and therefore the incidence and prevalence is likely to be different now.

A Taiwanese study (Lai and Tseng 2010) used a database of ICD-9 diagnostic codes to calculate myasthenia gravis incidence and prevalence rates in a very large population. Although formal validation was not performed, the included patients were verified against a "serious accidents and diseases" database, which required confirmation by a specialist. In the 2001–2007 study, incidence rates were 2.0–2.2 cases per 100 000 population per year and prevalence rates 14.0 per 100 000 population. Myasthenia gravis occurred in all age groups, with the highest incidence in older individuals and the lowest incidence in the 10- to 14-year-olds for both sexes.

The average incidence per million for both males and females was: 0.89 for children age 0–4 years; 0.69 for children age 5–9 years; and 0.37 for those between ages 10–14 years; and 0.83 in young people in the 15–19 age group.

The incidence was lowest in the 10- to 14-year age group and higher in the older age groups for both sexes. The incidence was significantly higher in females than in males in age groups of 0–4 and 15–54 years. The prevalence increased steadily from 8.4 per 100 000 in 2000 to 14.0 per 100 000 in 2007 (Lai and Tseng 2010).

African Studies

The only data available for African children is based on AChR-antibody-positive myasthenia gravis test results. This showed the annual incidence rate to be constant at 3 per million for children aged below 15 years of age (irrespective of pre or postpubertal onset) (Heckmann et al. 2012). Younger children developed ocular myasthenia gravis with a mean age at symptom onset of 5.1 years; older children developed generalised myasthenia gravis at mean age at onset 10.2 years.

Studies from Dar Es Salaam, Tanzania, for the period between 1988–1998 showed that the annual incidence of myasthenia gravis of both sexes was 3 per million population in all age groups. (Matuja et al. 2001). The incidence was lowest in those aged below 10 years. Incidence was higher in females. Studies revealed that 47% were ocular myasthenia and 53% were mild to moderately severe generalised myasthenia gravis. The authors concluded that myasthenia gravis is as rare in Tanzania as it is in other sub-Saharan countries.

South America

In a Brazilian study by Aguiar et al. between 1989 and 2009, 122 patients were identified; 85 (69.7%) females and 37 (30.3%) males. For children age under 12 years, there were five patients, all female; they all presented with generalised myasthenia gravis (Aguiar et al. 2010).

Slovakia

In a recent Slovakian study data from medical records of myasthenia gravis patients registered in Slovakia were analysed. The crude incidence increased from 0.36 per 100 000 in 1977–1989 to 1.74 per 100 000 in 2010–2015. The crude myasthenia gravis prevalence on 31 December 2015 was 24.75 per 100 000. The study concluded that the age at onset and incidence increased significantly over the study period due to marked increase of myasthenia gravis incidence in the elderly, particularly those over 70 years (Lavrnić et al. 2018).

CONCLUSIONS

There are few epidemiological studies of childhood myasthenia. Furthermore, there are hardly any studies that focus solely on the epidemiology of congenital myasthenia. The majority of studies are based on myasthenia gravis in the adult population. Where paediatric patients have been included in the adult studies, the age ranges have often been broadly defined with variability between studies; some include children up to 19 years old which one would argue classifies as being in the adult age range.

The highest quality studies show that childhood myasthenia is a rare condition with a mean incidence of antibody-positive autoimmune myasthenia of 1.5 per million children per year in the United Kingdom (Parr et al. 2014); the incidence and prevalence increase with age, into adolescence (9.2 per million children under 18 years of age). Most cases are of autoimmune myasthenia; congenital myasthenia is more common in young children. Prevalence of genetically confirmed CMS was 9.2 per million children under the age of 18 (Parr et al. 2014). There is variability in epidemiology between countries and across regions, in part due to study methods; however, genetic and environmental influences are likely to be relevant.

In the future, high quality population studies of myasthenia are required to confirm international similarities and differences in the incidence and prevalence of myasthenia, and whether the rates change with time.

REFERENCES

Aguiar AA, Carvalho AF, Costa CM et al. (2010) Myasthenia gravis in Ceará, Brazil: clinical and epidemiological aspects. *Arq Neuropsiquiatr* **68:** 843–848.

Aiello I, Pastorino M, Sotgiu S et al. (1997) Epidemiology of myasthenia gravis in northwestern Sardinia. *Neuroepidemiology* **16:** 199–206.

Breiner A, Widdifield J, Katzberg HD, Barnett C, Bril V, Tu K (2016) Epidemiology of myasthenia gravis in Ontario, Canada. *Neuromuscul Disord* **26:** 41–46.

Carr AS, Cardwell CR, McCarron PO, McConville J (2010) A systematic review of population based epidemiological studies in Myasthenia Gravis. *BMC Neurol* **10:** 46.

Casetta I, Fallica E, Govoni V, Azzini C, Tola M, Granieri E (2004) Incidence of myasthenia gravis in the province of Ferrara: a community-based study. *Neuroepidemiology* **23:** 281–284.

Chiu HC, Vincent A, Newsom-Davis J, Hsieh KH, Hung T (1987) Myasthenia gravis: population differences in disease expression and acetylcholine receptor antibody titers between Chinese and Caucasians. *Neurology* **37:** 1854–1857.

Christensen PB, Jensen TS, Tsiropoulos I et al. (1993) Incidence and prevalence of myasthenia gravis in western Denmark: 1975 to 1989. *Neurology* **43**: 1779–1783.

Emilia-Romagna Study Group on Clinical and Epidemiological Problems in Neurology (1998) Incidence of myasthenia gravis in the Emilia-Romagna region: a prospective multicenter study. *Neurology* **51**: 255–258.

Ferrari G, Lovaste MG (1992) Epidemiology of myasthenia gravis in the province of Trento (northern Italy). *Neuroepidemiology* **11**: 135–142.

Guidetti D, Sabadini R, Bondavalli M et al. (1998) Epidemiological study of myasthenia gravis in the province of Reggio Emilia, Italy. *Eur J Epidemiol* **14**: 381–387.

Guptill JT, Sanders DB, Evoli A (2011) Anti-MuSK antibody myasthenia gravis: clinical findings and response to treatment in two large cohorts. *Muscle Nerve* **44**: 36–40.

Heckmann JM, Hansen P, van Toorn R, Lubbe E, Jan van Rensburg E, Wilmhurst J (2012) The characteristics of juvenile myasthenia gravis among South Africans. *S Afr Med J* **102(6)**: 532–536.

Jacobson DL, Gange SJ, Rose NR, Graham NM (1997) Epidemiology and estimated population burden of selected autoimmune diseases in the United States. *Clin Immunol Immunopathol* **84**: 223–243.

Kalb B, Matell G, Pirskanen R, Lambe M (2002) Epidemiology of myasthenia gravis: a population-based study in Stockholm, Sweden. *Neuroepidemiology* **21**: 221–225.

Lai CH, Tseng HF (2010) Nationwide population-based epidemiological study of myasthenia gravis in Taiwan. *Neuroepidemiology* **35**: 66–71.

Lavrnić D, Jarebinski M, Rakocević-Stojanović V et al. (1999) Epidemiological and clinical characteristics of myasthenia gravis in Belgrade, Yugoslavia (1983–1992). *Acta Neurol Scand* **100**: 168–174.

Lavrnić D, Martinka I, Fulova M, Spalekova M, Spalek P (2018) Epidemiology of myasthenia gravis in Slovakia in the Years 1977–2015. *Neuroepidemiology* **50**: 153–159.

Matuja WB, Aris EA, Gabone J, Mgaya EM (2001) Incidence and characteristics of Myasthenia gravis in Dar Es Salaam, Tanzania. *East Afr Med J* **78**: 473–476.

Mombaur B, Lesosky MR, Liebenberg L, Vreede H, Heckmann JM (2015) Incidence of acetylcholine receptor antibody-positive myasthenia gravis in South Africa. *Muscle Nerve* **51**: 533–537.

Oöpik M, Kaasik AE, Jakobsen J (2003) A population based epidemiological study on myasthenia gravis in Estonia. *J Neurol Neurosurg Psychiatry* **74**: 1638–1643.

Parr JR, Andrew MJ, Finnis M, Beeson D, Vincent A, Jayawant S (2014) How common is childhood myasthenia? The UK incidence and prevalence of autoimmune and congenital myasthenia. *Arch Dis Child* **99**: 539–542.

Pedersen EG, Hallas J, Hansen K, Jensen PE, Gaist D (2013) Late onset myasthenia not on the increase: a nationwide register study in Denmark, 1996–2009. *Eur J Neurol* **20**: 309–314.

Phillips LH 2nd (2003) The epidemiology of myasthenia gravis. *Ann N Y Acad Sci* **998**: 407–412.

Popperud TH, Boldingh MI, Brunborg C et al. (2017) Juvenile myasthenia gravis in Norway: A nationwide epidemiological study. *Eur J Paediatr Neurol* **21(2)**: 312–317.

Poulas K, Tsibri E, Kokla A et al. (2001) Epidemiology of seropositive myasthenia gravis in Greece. *J Neurol Neurosurg Psychiatry* **71**: 352–356.

Radhakrishnan K, Thacker AK, Maloo JC, Gerryo SE, Mousa ME (1988) Descriptive epidemiology of some rare neurological diseases in Benghazi, Libya. *Neuroepidemiology* **7**: 159–164.

Wang W, Chen Y-P, Wang Z-K, Wei D-N, Yin L (2013) A cohort study on myasthenia gravis patients in China. *Neurol Sci* **34(10)**: 1759–1764.

Weatherbee SD, Anderson KV, Niswander LA (2006) LDL-receptor-related protein 4 is crucial for formation of the neuromuscular junction. *Development* **133**: 4993–5000.

Wong V, Hawkins BR, Yu YL (1992) Myasthenia gravis in Hong Kong Chinese. 2. Paediatric disease. *Acta Neurol Scand* **86**: 68–72.

Yu YL, Hawkins BR, Ip MSM, Wong V, Woo E (1992) Epidemiology and adult disease of Myasthenia gravis in Hong Kong Chinese. *Acta Neurol Scand* **86**: 113–119.

Zisimopoulou P, Evangelakou P, Tzartos J et al. (2014) A comprehensive analysis of the epidemiology and clinical characteristics of anti-LRP4 in myasthenia gravis. *J Autoimmun* **52**: 139–145.

Autoimmune Myasthenia in Children

Sithara Ramdas, Heinz Jungbluth

INTRODUCTION

Myasthenia gravis is an autoimmune disorder, predominantly caused by antibodies binding to the acetylcholine receptor (AChR) or functionally related proteins in the postsynaptic membrane at the neuromuscular junction (NMJ) (Phillips and Vincent 2016). There are four main forms of childhood myasthenia gravis, distinguished mainly by age at onset and variable clinical features, including transient neonatal myasthenia gravis (TNM), fetal acetylcholine receptor inactivation syndrome (FARIS), ocular myasthenia gravis (OMG) and juvenile myasthenia gravis (JMG). Although itself a rare disease with an incidence rate of 1–1.5/million population (Parr et al. 2014), JMG is the most frequent of the four forms and, according to most authors, defined by an onset before 18 years. Childhood myasthenia gravis must be distinguished from the genetically determined congenital myasthenic syndromes (CMS), the Lambert–Eaton Myasthenic Syndrome (LEMS) and other early-onset neuromuscular disorders with overlapping features.

PATHOPHYSIOLOGY

The principal pathophysiological mechanism is the same throughout different forms of childhood myasthenia gravis, and involves an antibody-mediated attack against postjunctional proteins involved in the acetylcholine (Ach) pathway, in particular the AChR, a sodium channel topping the junctional folds at the postjunctional end of the NMJ (Vincent et al. 2001, 2006; Phillips and Vincent 2016). The AChR is composed of five different subunits (α, β, γ, δ, ϵ), with important differences between the fetal (α, α, β, γ, δ) and the adult (α, α, β, δ, ϵ) receptor isoforms. AChR antibodies are predominantly IgG1 and IgG3 subclasses, with the ability to induce complement-mediated damage to the postsynaptic membrane, resulting in destruction and simplification of the NMJ, receptor endocytosis, and occasionally direct AChR block (Vincent 2002). There are other important elements of the postsynaptic NMJ that themselves may become the target of autoimmune attack, such as muscle-specific kinase (MuSK), and low-density lipoprotein receptor 4 (LRP4). MuSK, a postsynaptic protein critically implicated in NMJ development and maintenance, is activated through binding to LRP4, following LRP4 activation by agrin released from the presynaptic nerve terminal. This process leads to MuSK phosphorylation, ultimately resulting in the clustering of AChR and RAPSYN (Receptor-Associated Protein at the SYNaptic cleft) on top of postsynaptic folds, an event essential for efficient transmission at the NMJ (Kim et al. 2008). Anti-MuSK antibodies, a less common cause of myasthenia gravis, are IgG4 subclass antibodies which exert their pathogenic effect by preventing the interaction between MuSK and LRP4, thereby inhibiting agrin-dependent AChR clustering (Koneczny et al. 2013). Pathogenic antibodies against LRP4 of the complement-activating IgG1 type impeding agrin-induced AChR clustering have also been recently reported (Zisimopoulou et al. 2014).

EPIDEMIOLOGY

There are important epidemiological differences in autoimmune childhood myasthenia gravis depending on age at onset, sex and ethnicity. In prepubertal children with myasthenia gravis, there is an equal sex ratio, except for in Afro-Caribbean children where there is a female preponderance (Andrews et al. 1994; Evoli et al. 1998). Compared to the postpubertal group, prepubertal children are also more commonly seronegative (36–50% vs <10% of cases) (Andrews et al. 1994), have a higher incidence of OMG and higher remission rates (Evoli et al. 1998; Batocchi et al. 1990). The characteristics of postpubertal myasthenia gravis are similar to adult-onset myasthenia gravis with higher female preponderance, higher rates of generalised myasthenia gravis and lower rates of remission (Batocchi et al. 1990; Andrews et al. 1994). In general, JMG is more common in oriental populations (Chiu et al. 1987; Kawaguchi et al. 2004; Zhang et al. 2007) and Afro-Caribbean children (Andrews et al. 1994). In the Chinese and Japanese population, paediatric presentations account for 50% of all myasthenia gravis cases compared to 10–15% in the Caucasian population (Phillips et al. 1992). Overall, JMG is also a milder disease in the oriental population, with predominantly OMG and lower rates of generalisation (Chiu et al. 1987; Kawaguchi et al. 2004; Zhang et al. 2007). Afro-Caribbean children have been reported to have a more treatment resistant form of OMG (Heckmann et al. 2007). In terms of sex differences, boys, across all ages have milder disease and higher rates of remission (Andrews et al. 1994).

TRANSIENT NEONATAL MYASTHENIA GRAVIS AND THE FETAL AChR INACTIVATION SYNDROME

TNMG (Papazian 1992), caused by placental transfer of maternal antibodies, aff around 10–15% of infants born to mothers with AChR-related myasthenia gravis (Vernet-der Garabedian et al. 1994) and, less frequently, MuSK-related myasthenia gravis (Niks et al. 2008; Béhin et al. 2008). Symptoms comprise variable hypotonia, feeding difficulties and respiratory impairment, occasionally necessitating tube feeding, ventilatory support and intermittent medical treatment. Whilst TNMG is usually a self-limiting condition resolving within weeks or months, another early-onset form of myasthenia gravis with persistent features due to maternal antibodies against the fetal AChR isoform has been recently described, termed fetal acetylcholine receptor inactivation syndrome (or fetal AChR inactivation syndrome; FARIS) (Oskoui et al. 2008; Hacohen et al. 2014; Allen et al. 2016). FARIS is characterised by clinical features ranging from potentially fatal arthrogryposis multiplex congenita (AMC) to a mild, predominantly facial and bulbar myopathy. Mothers of aff infants usually have myasthenic symptoms but may be asymptomatic, and, as in TNMG (Téllez-Zenteno et al. 2004), there appears to some correlation between the degree of maternal treatment and neonatal outcome. Whilst aff infants do not appear to respond as well to acetylcholine esterase (AChE) inhibition and/or immunoglobulins (see Management section), probably reflective of structural damage that has already occurred in utero, some benefit of salbutamol has been recently reported (Allen et al. 2016).

JUVENILE MYASTHENIA GRAVIS

Fatigable muscle weakness is the hallmark of JMG. The muscle weakness can be generalised or localised, is usually more proximal than distal and nearly always includes eye muscles, with prominent ptosis, ophthalmoplegia and diplopia (Andrews 2004; Parr and Jayawant 2007). Most children with JMG have eye involvement at presentation, often unilateral or asymmetric (Mullaney et al. 2000; Kupersmith and Ying 2005), and in 10–20% of cases this may remain the only sign (Rodríguez et al. 1983; Andrews 2004; Ashraf et al. 2006). Bulbar involvement may also be a presenting feature. The weakness typically varies from day to day and over the course of a day, sometimes with normal muscle strength, particularly in the morning. Disease onset can be insidious or acute during an intercurrent illness. With more insidious presentations, children may have had unrecognised symptoms for weeks or months, including intermittent double vision, chewing and swallowing difficulties, and/or unexplained physical problems, particularly in the evening. The diagnosis of myasthenia gravis in very young children may be particularly challenging because of its rarity and often subtle features. A myasthenic crisis (Bershad et al. 2008), either spontaneously or during intercurrent illness, may result in severe profound weakness affecting skeletal, bulbar and respiratory muscles and can be life-threatening if not recognised promptly and treated as an emergency.

JMG due to MuSK antibodies is more common in teenage girls (Pasnoor et al. 2010). There is predominant bulbar involvement with facial weakness and tongue wasting (Evoli et al. 2003; Farrugia et al. 2007). An associated ocular phenotype is also now well recognised (Evoli et al. 2017; Lee and Jander 2017).

Myasthenia gravis due to LRP4 antibodies is rare and felt to affect a predominantly female cohort with mainly ocular and only mild generalised involvement (Zisimopoulou et al. 2014).

OCULAR MYASTHENIA GRAVIS

In OMG there is exclusive extra-ocular muscle weakness at presentation, the disease remains restricted to the eyes and, per definition, generalised muscle weakness does not follow within 2 years of onset (Mullaney et al. 2000; Kupersmith et al. 2003; Luchanok and Kaminski 2008). The diagnostic criteria for paediatric OMG have been suggested by several authors (Kupersmith et al. 2003; Pineles et al. 2010). OMG is seen in 10–15% of childhood autoimmune myasthenia (Andrews 2004), with a higher prevalence in oriental population (Chiu et al. 1987; Wong et al. 1992; Kawaguchi et al. 2004; Zhang et al. 2007). The rate of subsequent generalisation varies between 8% and 43% (Mullaney et al. 2000; McCreery et al. 2002; Kim et al. 2003; Ortiz and Borchert 2008; Pineles et al. 2010) compared to 80% in adult myasthenia gravis (Kalb et al. 2002), with the lowest rates of generalisation in prepubertal and oriental children. The remission rate varies between 13% and 50% (Mullaney et al. 2000; McCreery et al. 2002; Kim et al. 2003; Ortiz and Borchert 2008; Pineles et al. 2010). Children with OMG (and those with generalised JMG where ocular involvement is prominent) especially under the age of 8 years are at risk of amblyopia (3–10%), therefore regular ophthalmology review is essential to ensure maintenance of the visual axis and preservation of binocular vision.

INVESTIGATIONS

The diagnosis of myasthenia gravis rests on the detection of causative antibodies, neurophysiological evidence of a neuromuscular transmission defect and/or a positive response to AChE inhibitors in the context of suggestive clinical features. Ancillary investigations such as thymus imaging are important to exclude an associated thymoma.

Antibodies

The presence of specific antibodies to the AChR, MuSK and LRP4 is diagnostic. The small proportion of cases where no antibodies are identified on standard assays are termed seronegative myasthenia gravis (SNMG).

AChR ANTIBODIES

The anti-AChR radio immunoassay (RIA) is the standard assay, with a positivity of 40–70% in ocular and of 85% to 95% in generalised myasthenia gravis (Vincent and Newsom-Davis 1985; Sommer et al. 1993). Cell-based cluster AChR assays introduced more recently (Leite et al. 2008) have a crucial role in SNMG patients. In general, the proportion of SNMG patients with antibodies to clustered AChR ranges from 16% to 60% (Leite et al. 2008; Jacob et al. 2012; Devic et al. 2014; Rodríguez Cruz et al. 2015). The cluster AChR assay is particularly important in paediatric myasthenia gravis, with higher rates of cluster AChR assay positivity in pre-pubertal disease onset SNMG children and in the OMG group, with milder disease and higher rates of remission (Rodríguez Cruz et al. 2015).

MuSK ANTIBODIES

MuSK antibodies have been reported in around 40% of SNMG patients in the adult Caucasian population, with a wide range (0–70%) likely related to ethnicity (Hoch et al. 2001; Scuderi et al. 2002; Sanders et al. 2003; Vincent et al. 2005; Padua et al. 2006; Chang et al. 2009; Guptill et al. 2011). The use of a cell-based assay detected anti-MuSK antibodies in 8% of SNMG patients (Rodríguez Cruz et al. 2015); however, another international study of analysing serum from SNMG patients using a similar assay suggested that those antibodies were IgM antibodies, of uncertain relevance in myasthenia gravis (Tsonis et al. 2015).

LRP4 ANTIBODIES

LRP4 antibodies have been reported in several SNMG cases, with a highly variable detection rate between 3% and 54%, depending on ethnicity, and different antigens and assays used (Higuchi et al. 2011; Pevzner et al. 2012; Zhang et al. 2012; Zisimopoulou et al. 2014). Double positivity for antibodies to LRP4 and AChR and MuSK and LRP4 has been reported and will require further exploration (Zisimopoulou et al. 2014).

Neurophysiology

Repetitive nerve stimulation (RNS) to detect an electrical decrement of more than 10% in the amplitude of the negative peak of the compound muscle action potential is one of the useful diagnostic tests. The maximal decrement is measured at the third to fifth response, on supramaximal repetitive (3–20Hz) nerve stimulation. RNS when done in the orbicularis oculi during stimulation of the facial nerve and single fibre electromyography (SFEMG) has a sensitivity of 78% and 96.4%, respectively (Sarrigiannis et al. 2006; Zambelis et al. 2011). Both RNS and SFEMG can be technically challenging in young children. Stimulated single fibre EMG (sSFEMG), an adaptation of classic SFEMG, is better tolerated in children and does not require patient co-operation (Pitt 2008).

The Tensilon test (Osserman and Teng 1956) involves intravenous administration of a short-acting cholinesterase inhibitor (edrophonium chloride) under controlled conditions. In patients with myasthenia gravis, a rapid but short-lived (5–30 minutes) improvement in ptosis and/or muscle strength is expected shortly after injection. In addition to a careful clinical observation, video recording pre- and post-tensilon are useful to document objective improvement of ptosis or muscle power. With a view to potentially life-threatening cholinergic side effects, full resuscitation equipment and atropine should be readily available. Positive results can be seen in up to 90% of JMG patients but the tensilon test has low specificity and should not be the only basis for diagnosis (Afifi and Bell 1993).

Thymus Imaging

Although thymoma is rare in JMG (Chiang et al. 2009) compared to adult myasthenia gravis, the thymus must be imaged either by computed tomography or MRI once the diagnosis of JMG has been established. Thymus hyperplasia is the commonest abnormality of the thymus in AChR–associated JMG (Chiang et al. 2009) and often confirmed histologically post-thymectomy. Thymus hyperplasia and germinal centre B cell alterations are not a common feature of MuSK-associated myasthenia gravis and OMG but have been documented in SNMG patients (Hayashi et al. 2007).

MANAGEMENT

The overall management of JMG must be under direction of a paediatric neurologist who may seek advice from a paediatric myasthenia gravis or neuromuscular specialist as required. Most children will require a multi-disciplinary team of professionals, including a general and community paediatrician, ophthalmologist, physiotherapist, occupational therapist, speech and language therapist and specialist nurses. There are recent national and international guidelines concerning the management of myasthenia gravis in adults (Skeie et al. 2006; Sussman et al. 2015; Sanders et al. 2016). As the underlying pathophysiology is essentially the same, treatment strategies in JMG have been largely extrapolated from studies concerning adult myasthenia gravis. Table 5.1 illustrates a overview of JMG treatment. The main treatment options include AChE inhibitors, immunosuppressive therapy with steroids and/or other immunosuppressive agents,

Table 5.1 Main characteristics of the four principal forms of childhood myasthenia gravis

	FARIS	TNMG	JMG		OMG
Onset	Antenatal	Neonatal	2–18 years		>2 years
Antibodies	AChR (fetal)	AChR (adult) (MuSK)	AChR (MuSK) (LRP4)		AChR (MuSK)
Clinical features			*Infancy onset*	*Childhood onset*	
Hypotonia	+++	+++	+++	+	−
Weakness	++	++	+++	++	−
Ocular	+	++	++	+++	+++
Bulbar	++	++	+++	++	−
Respiratory	++	++	++	+	−
Others	AMC, VPI	Pyloric stenosis	Rarely thymoma		
Management[a]	Supportive Pyridostigmine Neostigmine (IVIG) Salbutamol	Supportive Pyridostigmine Neostigmine (IVIG, PLEX)	Pyridostigmine Corticosteroids Steroid-sparing agents (IVIG, PLEX) (Thymectomy)		Pyridostigmine (Corticosteroids)

[a]Brackets indicate rarely used second-line treatment.
FARIS, fetal acetylcholine receptor inactivation syndrome; TNMG, transient neonatal myasthenia gravis; JMG, juvenile myasthenia gravis; OMG, ocular myasthenia gravis; AChR, acetylcholine receptor; MuSK, muscle-specific kinase; LRP4, low-density lipoprotein receptor-related protein 4; AMC, arthrogryposis multiplex congenita; VPI, velopharyngeal insufficiency; IVIG, intravenous immunoglobulin; PLEX, plasmapheresis. +++ = very common, ++ = common, + = occasionally observed.

thymectomy and/or a combination of the above. Advice regarding precautions during surgery and/or general anaesthesia, intercurrent illness and avoidance of contraindicated medications should also be part of a comprehensive JMG management. In addition, during acute crises intravenous immunoglobulins, steroids or plasma exchange may be needed.

Acetylcholinesterase Inhibitors

AChE inhibitors are the first-line of treatment. They increase the half-life of acetylcholine thus indirectly prolonging its actions at the synaptic cleft. Pyridostigmine (Mestinon) is commonly used because of its better side effect profile and longer duration of action compared with neostigmine. The initial dose for pyridostigmine is 0.5–1mg/kg every 4–6 hours in smaller children, up to 30–60mg every 4–6 hours in adolescents, followed by gradual increases depending on clinical response. Doses above 7mg/kg/day (or 360mg/day in older teenagers) are unlikely to add any beneficial effects and there are concerns regarding potential adverse effects on the postsynaptic membrane. A pyridostigmine slow-release formulation (Mestinon Timespan) is available and may be administered at night in children who have pronounced weakness first thing in the morning, but dose adjustments can be challenging due to variable absorption. Neostigmine can be administered intramuscularly or intravenously, making it suitable in acute or perioperative settings, and/or in infants with TNMG. Side effects of AChE inhibitors are mainly due to muscarinic effects at high doses and include abdominal cramps, diarrhoea, hypersalivation, miosis and bradycardia; if those are pronounced but the treatment effect is good, introduction of an antimuscarinic agent such as propantheline may be warranted. Discontinuation of AChE treatment under close observation ought to be considered in children with acute worsening of symptoms on higher doses, as a cholinergic crisis can cause severe muscle weakness, mimicking a myasthenic crisis.

Except for some patient with OMG, most patients with JMG will require additional treatment and prolonged treatment trials beyond 2–3 weeks without response are thus not justifiable. Patients with MuSK-related myasthenia gravis are less likely to respond to AChE inhibitors, and some may even demonstrate clinical worsening and significant side effects (Sanders et al. 2003; Guptill et al. 2011).

Immunosuppression and/or Immunomodulatory Treatment

Immunosuppression and/or immunomodulatory treatment includes various options:

- **Corticosteroids** are the most commonly used first-line immunosuppressive therapy with an initial response in up to 80% of patients. A response is usually seen within 2–3 weeks but may take up to a couple of months (Batocchi et al. 1990). There are two main regimes for initiating treatment, a slow low dose escalation and rapid high dose escalation. The rapid high dose escalation usually leads to a quick response but carries a risk of clinical worsening, typically in the first week but sometimes later (Ionita and Acsadi 2013), and should thus be initiated in hospital, up to a maximum dose of usually 1.5mg/kg on alternate days. Once a response to treatment has been observed, the high dosage can be reduced by 5mg every 4–6 months, initially to 1mg/kg on alternate days for 4–6 months. Further reductions should then be much slower, for example by 5mg every month up to 20mg alternate days, then by 1mg every couple of months. A proportion of patients may require low dose steroids for several years. In acute settings, intravenous methylprednisolone may play a role if the patient does not respond adequately to plasmapheresis alone (Chang et al. 2009). As with other conditions requiring long-term steroid treatment, substantial side effects including weight gain, poor growth, hypertension, hyperglycaemia, behavioural concerns, osteoporosis, infection risk and cushingoid features have to be anticipated and monitored for.

- *Steroid-sparing agents* are used in isolation in those who fail to respond to corticosteroids, or as an adjunct in those who are long-term steroid dependent with significant side effects.
- *Azathioprine* is a well-established and effective treatment in both adult and JMG (Evoli et al. 1998; Palace et al. 1998; Mullaney et al. 2000; Ashraf et al. 2006). It inhibits purine metabolism and affects rapidly dividing cells, including lymphocytes, and thiopurine methyltransferase (TPMT) activity must be checked prior to therapy initiation to identify patients at highest risk for myelosuppression where lower doses need to be used. The usual initial dose in children is 1mg/kg/day, followed by increments of 0.5mg/kg/day every month up to a maximum of 2.5mg/kg/day. The usual initial adolescent and adult dose is 50mg daily, increased by 50mg every 4 weeks to a maximum of 150–200mg daily. Azathioprine may take 3–12 months before an improvement becomes evident. Regular blood count and liver function monitoring is required, considering side effects including dose-dependent bone marrow suppression, gastro-intestinal symptoms, reversible hepatitis and/or (rarely) pancreatitis, as well as hypersensitivity reactions. There is a small long-term risk of malignancy.
- *Mycophenolate mofetil (MMF)* impairs purine synthesis and inhibits the proliferation of B and T lymphocytes. Despite promising results in retrospective studies (Chaudhry et al. 2001; Meriggioli et al. 2003), a randomised, double-blinded trial investigating MMF vs placebo as a steroid-sparing agent in adult myasthenia gravis patients showed no clear differences in symptom reduction or achievement of pharmacological remission (Sanders et al. 2008). In JMG, it may be considered if other therapies are ineffective or not tolerated, but its teratogenic potential has to be considered in females of child-bearing age.
- *Rituximab* is a chimeric monoclonal antibody against the B lymphocyte antigen CD20. CD20 regulates the early steps of cell-cycle initiation and is involved in activation, differentiation, and growth of B-lymphocytes. Rituximab produces a substantial reduction in circulating CD20 B-cells for up to 6 months and at times longer (McLaughlin et al. 1998; Edwards et al. 2004). There is multiple evidence of its effectiveness in treatment-refractory myasthenia gravis, in particular the MuSK-related form (Wylam et al. 2003; Maddison et al. 2011; Koul et al. 2012; Anderson et al. 2016; Tandan et al. 2017; Hehir et al. 2017). The dose is usually 375mg/m^2 weekly for 4 weeks, with standardised blood monitoring regimes pre- and post-rituximab. Side effects include allergic reactions during the infusion, headaches, and risk of infections.
- *Intravenous immunoglobulin (IVIG)* is an effective treatment option in JMG (Selcen et al. 2000; Zinman and Bril 2008), in particular in younger children where plasma exchange can be technically challenging. In acute settings, the total dose is 2g/kg, given either over 2 days (as 1g/kg/day) or 5 days (as 0.4g/kg/day). IVIG can also be used as a maintenance therapy, whilst initiating steroid-sparing agents, or if steroids/steroid-sparing agents have been ineffective or not tolerated. Side effects include allergic reactions, headaches, flu-like illness, aseptic meningitis, and, rarely, nephrotoxicity. As with other blood products, IVIG also carries the risk of blood borne disease transmission.
- *Plasma exchange (PLEX)* aims to remove circulating antibodies and, like IVIG, is helpful in acute situations (Batocchi et al. 1990) or prior to thymectomy. Five cycles of exchange are usually performed every other day but can be performed daily during a myasthenic crisis. Clinical improvement is usually seen within days. Limiting factors include availability in the specific hospital setting, and appropriate venous access which may be an issue in small children. Complications include sepsis, hypotension and pulmonary embolism. The effects of PLEX are transient, and repeat cycles are usually required 2–4 weekly if used as a medium or long-term treatment option.
- *Thymectomy* has been well recognised as an important treatment option in the management of JMG and has recently also been the topic of a randomised trial in adults (Wolfe et al. 2016). In children, the rate of remission after thymectomy is higher (16–67%) than the rate of spontaneous remission (15–45%) (Rodríguez et al. 1983; Andrews 1998; Skeie et al. 2006). The general consensus is that

thymectomy is indicated in peri- and postpubertal children with moderate to severe AChR-related myasthenia gravis (Andrews 1998; Evoli et al. 1998) but it may also be considered and be effective in prepubertal children (Heng et al. 2014) if medical treatment is unsuccessful. Early thymectomy (performed within the first year after symptom onset) appears to be associated with higher remission rates than late thymectomy (Rodríguez et al. 1983; Adams et al. 1990; Andrews 1998; Seybold 1998). The effects of thymectomy can take several months to 2 years to be evident (Lakhoo et al. 1997; Tracy et al. 2009). Thymectomy is mandatory if a thymoma is present, but this is very rare in children. In childhood myasthenia, the role of thymectomy in settings other than JMG is controversial. Although not a typical indication, better remission rates and lesser frequent generalisation has been reported in small series of paediatric OMG patients treated with thymectomy (Ortiz and Borchert 2008; Pineles et al. 2010). Thymectomy seems to be of little benefit in MuSK-related myasthenia gravis compared to AChR-related myasthenia gravis. The role of thymectomy in seronegative patients needs careful thought, considering that a proportion of this group may have a genetic form of myasthenia.

A practical management flowchart for autoimmune myasthenia gravis in children is presented in Figure 5.1.

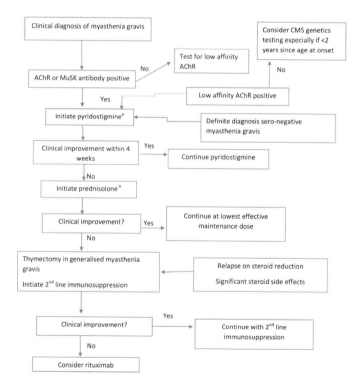

Figure 5.1   Myasthenia gravis treatment flowchart. [a]Use with caution in sero-negative myasthenia gravis if CMS genetics, in particular DOK7 and COLQ, are not available due to risk of clinical deterioration.

[b]In myasthenia gravis, slow dose prednisolone escalation can take up to 3–6 months to be efficacious. If moderate to severe myasthenia gravis symptoms at presentation, consider rapid in-hospital prednisolone escalation, and IVIG or PLEX to control symptoms whilst awaiting response to prednisolone.

AChR, acetylcholine receptor; CMS, congenital myasthenic syndromes; IVIG, intravenous immunoglobulin; MuSK, muscle-specific kinase; PLEX, plasmapheresis.

SUPPORTIVE MANAGEMENT AND PRECAUTIONS

Medications

Certain medications are known to worsen myasthenic symptoms and ought to be avoided, including antibiotics such as aminoglycosides, tetracyclines and fluoroquinolones; cardiac agents such as quinidine and beta-blockers; and neuromuscular blocking agents. Health professionals looking after JMG patients must refer to a formulary or prescribing database to ensure that any new medication is safe to use in myasthenia gravis.

Surgery and Anaesthesia

When patients with myasthenia gravis require surgery, where possible neuromuscular blockade agents must be avoided. If required, polarising agents (e.g. succinylcholine) are preferred over non-depolarising agents (e.g. rocuronium and vecuronium).

Infections

Children with JMG can deteriorate very quickly during acute illness, due to infection-related immune responses which can aggravate myasthenic symptoms and/or side effects of immunosuppressive treatment.

PROGNOSIS

JMG is a relatively rare but serious treatable condition which can be life-threatening. Deaths have been reported in the past but should be avoidable with prompt diagnosis and appropriate management. Compared to adults where the remission rates are less than 10%, spontaneous remission rates in JMG range from 15% to 34.7% (Rodríguez et al. 1983; Andrews et al. 1994; Evoli et al. 1998; Ashraf et al. 2006), and are highest in prepubertal and Caucasian children (Andrews et al. 1994).

CONCLUSIONS

Juvenile and other forms of childhood myasthenia gravis are rare but important conditions that ought to be recognised promptly to institute timely and effective treatments. Although the pathophysiology and principles are similar to those of adult forms, there are important differences that ought to be taken into consideration.

REFERENCES

Adams C, Theodorescu D, Murphy EG, Shandling B (1990) Thymectomy in juvenile myasthenia gravis. *J Child Neurol* **5:** 215–218.

Afifi AK, Bell WE (1993) Tests for juvenile myasthenia gravis: comparative diagnostic yield and prediction of outcome. *J Child Neurol* **8:** 403–411.

Allen NM, Hacohen Y, Palace J, Beeson D, Vincent A, Jungbluth H (2016) Salbutamol-responsive fetal acetylcholine receptor inactivation syndrome. *Neurology* **86:** 692–694.

Anderson D, Phan C, Johnston WS, Siddiqi ZA (2016) Rituximab in refractory myasthenia gravis: a prospective, open-label study with long-term follow-up. *Ann Clin Transl Neurol* **3:** 552–555.

Andrews PI (1998) A treatment algorithm for autoimmune myasthenia gravis in childhood. *Ann N Y Acad Sci* **841:** 789–802.

Andrews PI (2004) Autoimmune myasthenia gravis in childhood. *Semin Neurol* **24:** 101–110.

Andrews PI, Massey JM, Howard JF Jr, Sanders DB (1994) Race, sex, and puberty influence onset, severity, and outcome in juvenile myasthenia gravis. *Neurology* **44:** 1208–1214.

Ashraf VV, Taly AB, Veerendrakumar M, Rao S (2006) Myasthenia gravis in children: a longitudinal study. *Acta Neurol Scand* **114:** 119–123.

Batocchi AP, Evoli A, Palmisani MT, Lo Monaco M, Bartoccioni M, Tonali P (1990) Early-onset myasthenia gravis: clinical characteristics and response to therapy. *Eur J Pediatr* **150:** 66–68.

Béhin A, Mayer M, Kassis-Makhoul B et al. (2008) Severe neonatal myasthenia due to maternal anti-MuSK antibodies. *Neuromuscul Disord* **18:** 443–446.

Bershad EM, Feen ES, Suarez JI (2008) Myasthenia gravis crisis. *South Med J* **101:** 63–69.

Chang T, Gunaratne P, Gamage R, Riffsy MT, Vincent A (2009) MuSK-antibody-positive myasthenia gravis in a South Asian population. *J Neurol Sci* **284:** 33–35.

Chaudhry V, Cornblath DR, Griffin JW, O'Brien R, Drachman DB (2001) Mycophenolate mofetil: a safe and promising immunosuppressant in neuromuscular diseases. *Neurology* **56:** 94–96.

Chiang LM, Darras BT, Kang PB (2009) Juvenile myasthenia gravis. *Muscle Nerve* **39:** 423–431.

Chiu HC, Vincent A, Newsom-Davis J, Hsieh KH, Hung T (1987) Myasthenia gravis: population differences in disease expression and acetylcholine receptor antibody titers between Chinese and Caucasians. *Neurology* **37:** 1854–1857.

Devic P, Petiot P, Simonet T et al. (2014) Antibodies to clustered acetylcholine receptor: expanding the phenotype. *Eur J Neurol* **21:** 130–134.

Edwards JC, Leandro MJ, Cambridge G (2004) B lymphocyte depletion therapy with rituximab in rheumatoid arthritis. *Rheum Dis Clin North Am* **30:** 393–403, viii.

Evoli A, Batocchi AP, Bartoccioni E, Lino MM, Minisci C, Tonali P (1998) Juvenile myasthenia gravis with prepubertal onset. *Neuromuscul Disord* **8:** 561–567.

Evoli A, Tonali PA, Padua L et al. (2003) Clinical correlates with anti-MuSK antibodies in generalized seronegative myasthenia gravis. *Brain* **126:** 2304–2311.

Evoli A, Alboini PE, Iorio R, Damato V, Bartoccioni E (2017) Pattern of ocular involvement in myasthenia gravis with MuSK antibodies. *J Neurol Neurosurg Psychiatry* **88:** 761–763.

Farrugia ME, Kennett RP, Hilton-Jones D, Newsom-Davis J, Vincent A (2007) Quantitative EMG of facial muscles in myasthenia patients with MuSK antibodies. *Clin Neurophysiol* **118:** 269–277.

Guptill JT, Sanders DB, Evoli A (2011) Anti-MuSK antibody myasthenia gravis: clinical findings and response to treatment in two large cohorts. *Muscle Nerve* **44(1):** 36–40.

Hacohen Y, Jacobson LW, Byrne S et al. (2014) Fetal acetylcholine receptor inactivation syndrome: A myopathy due to maternal antibodies. *Neurol Neuroimmunol Neuroinflamm* **2(1):** e57.

Hayashi A, Shiono H, Ohta M, Ohta K, Okumura M, Sawa Y (2007) Heterogeneity of immunopathological features of AChR/MuSK autoantibody-negative myasthenia gravis. *J Neuroimmunol* **189:** 163–168.

Heckmann JM, Owen EP, Little F (2007) Myasthenia gravis in South Africans: racial differences in clinical manifestations. *Neuromuscul Disord* **17:** 929–934.

Hehir MK, Hobson-Webb LD, Benatar M et al. (2017) Rituximab as treatment for anti-MuSK myasthenia gravis: multicenter blinded prospective review. *Neurology* **89:** 1069–1077.

Heng HS, Lim M, Absoud M et al. (2014) Outcome of children with acetylcholine receptor (AChR) antibody positive juvenile myasthenia gravis following thymectomy. *Neuromuscul Disord* **24:** 25–30.

Higuchi O, Hamuro J, Motomura M, Yamanashi Y (2011) Autoantibodies to low-density lipoprotein receptor-related protein 4 in myasthenia gravis. *Ann Neurol* **69:** 418–422.

Hoch W, McConville J, Helms S, Newsom-Davis J, Melms A, Vincent A (2001) Auto-antibodies to the receptor tyrosine kinase MuSK in patients with myasthenia gravis without acetylcholine receptor antibodies. *Nat Med* **7:** 365–368.

Ionita CM, Acsadi G (2013) Management of juvenile myasthenia gravis. *Pediatr Neurol* **48:** 95–104.

Jacob S, Viegas S, Leite MI, Webster R, Cossins J, Kennett R et al. (2012) Presence and pathogenic relevance of antibodies to clustered acetylcholine receptor in ocular and generalized myasthenia gravis. *Arch Neurol* **69:** 994–1001.

Kalb B, Matell G, Pirskanen R, Lambe M (2002) Epidemiology of myasthenia gravis: a population-based study in Stockholm, Sweden. *Neuroepidemiology* **21:** 221–225.

Kawaguchi N, Kuwabara S, Nemoto Y et al. (2004) Treatment and outcome of myasthenia gravis: retrospective multi-center analysis of 470 Japanese patients, 1999–2000. *J Neurol Sci* **224:** 43–47.

Kim JH, Hwang JM, Hwang YS, Kim KJ, Chae J (2003) Childhood ocular myasthenia gravis. *Ophthalmology* **110:** 1458–1462.

Kim N, Stiegler AL, Cameron TO et al. (2008) Lrp4 is a receptor for agrin and forms a complex with MuSK. *Cell* **135:** 334–342.

Koneczny I, Cossins J, Waters P, Beeson D, Vincent A (2013) MuSK myasthenia gravis IgG4 disrupts the interaction of LRP4 with MuSK but both IgG4 and IgG1–3 can disperse preformed agrin-independent AChR clusters. *PLoS One* **8:** e80695.

Koul R, Al Futaisi A, Abdwani R (2012) Rituximab in severe seronegative juvenile myasthenia gravis: review of the literature. *Pediatr Neurol* **47:** 209–212.

Kupersmith MJ, Ying G (2005) Ocular motor dysfunction and ptosis in ocular myasthenia gravis: effects of treatment. *Br J Ophthalmol* **89:** 1330–1334.

Kupersmith MJ, Latkany R, Homel P (2003) Development of generalized disease at 2 years in patients with ocular myasthenia gravis. *Arch Neurol* **60:** 243–248.

Lakhoo K, De Fonseca J, Rodda J, Davies MRQ (1997) Thymectomy in black children with juvenile myasthenia gravis. *Pediatr Surg Int* **12:** 113–115.

Lee JI, Jander S (2017) Myasthenia gravis: recent advances in immunopathology and therapy. *Expert Rev Neurother* **17:** 287–299.

Leite MI, Jacob S, Viegas S et al. (2008) IgG1 antibodies to acetylcholine receptors in 'seronegative' myasthenia gravis. *Brain* **131:** 1940–1952.

Luchanok U, Kaminski HJ (2008) Ocular myasthenia: diagnostic and treatment recommendations and the evidence base. *Curr Opin Neurol* **21:** 8–15.

Maddison P, McConville J, Farrugia ME et al. (2011) The use of rituximab in myasthenia gravis and Lambert–Eaton myasthenic syndrome. *J Neurol Neurosurg Psychiatry* **82:** 671–673.

McCreery KM, Hussein MA, Lee AG, Paysse EA, Chandran R, Coats DK (2002) Major review: the clinical spectrum of pediatric myasthenia gravis: blepharoptosis, ophthalmoplegia and strabismus. A report of 14 cases. *Binocul Vis Strabismus Q* **17:** 181–186.

McLaughlin P, Grillo-López AJ, Link BK et al. (1998) Rituximab chimeric anti-CD20 monoclonal antibody therapy for relapsed indolent lymphoma: half of patients respond to a four-dose treatment program. *J Clin Oncol* **16:** 2825–2833.

Meriggioli MN, Ciafaloni E, Al-Hayk KA et al. (2003) Mycophenolate mofetil for myasthenia gravis: an analysis of efficacy, safety, and tolerability. *Neurology* **61:** 1438–1440.

Mullaney P, Vajsar J, Smith R, Buncic JR (2000) The natural history and ophthalmic involvement in childhood myasthenia gravis at the hospital for sick children. *Ophthalmology* **107:** 504–510.

Niks EH, Verrips A, Semmekrot BA et al. (2008) A transient neonatal myasthenic syndrome with anti-musk antibodies. *Neurology* **70:** 1215–1216.

Ortiz S, Borchert M (2008) Long-term outcomes of pediatric ocular myasthenia gravis. *Ophthalmology* **115(7):** 1245–1248.e1.

Oskoui M, Jacobson L, Chung WK et al. (2008) Fetal acetylcholine receptor inactivation syndrome and maternal myasthenia gravis. *Neurology* **71:** 2010–2012.

Osserman KE, Teng P (1956) Studies in myasthenia gravis – a rapid diagnostic test; further progress with edrophonium (tensilon) chloride. *J Am Med Assoc* **160:** 153–155.

Padua L, Tonali P, Aprile I, Caliandro P, Bartoccioni E, Evoli A (2006) Seronegative myasthenia gravis: comparison of neurophysiological picture in MuSK+ and MuSK- patients. *Eur J Neurol* **13:** 273–276.

Palace J, Newsom-Davis J, Lecky B, Myasthenia Gravis Study Group (1998) A randomized double-blind trial of prednisolone alone or with azathioprine in myasthenia gravis. *Neurology* **50:** 1778–1783.

Papazian O (1992) Transient neonatal myasthenia gravis. *J Child Neurol* **7:** 135–141.

Parr JR, Jayawant S (2007) Childhood myasthenia: clinical subtypes and practical management. *Dev Med Child Neurol* **49:** 629–635.

Parr JR, Andrew MJ, Finnis M, Beeson D, Vincent A, Jayawant S (2014) How common is childhood myasthenia? The UK incidence and prevalence of autoimmune and congenital myasthenia. *Arch Dis Child* **99:** 539–542.

Pasnoor M, Wolfe GI, Nations S et al. (2010) Clinical findings in MuSK-antibody positive myasthenia gravis: a U.S. experience. *Muscle Nerve* **41:** 370–374.

Pevzner A, Schoser B, Peters K et al. (2012) Anti-LRP4 autoantibodies in AChR- and MuSK-antibody-negative myasthenia gravis. *J Neurol* **259:** 427–435.

Phillips WD, Vincent A (2016) Pathogenesis of myasthenia gravis: update on disease types, models, and mechanisms. *F1000 Res* **5:** 5.

Phillips LH II, Torner JC, Anderson MS, Cox GM (1992) The epidemiology of myasthenia gravis in central and western Virginia. *Neurology* **42:** 1888–1893.

Pineles SL, Avery RA, Moss HE et al. (2010) Visual and systemic outcomes in pediatric ocular myasthenia gravis. *Am J Ophthalmol* **150(4):** 453–459.e3.

Pitt M (2008) Neurophysiological strategies for the diagnosis of disorders of the neuromuscular junction in children. *Dev Med Child Neurol* **50:** 328–333.

Rodríguez M, Gomez MR, Howard FM Jr, Taylor WF (1983) Myasthenia gravis in children: long-term follow-up. *Ann Neurol* **13:** 504–510.

Rodríguez Cruz PM, Al-Hajjar M, Huda S et al. (2015) Clinical features and diagnostic usefulness of antibodies to clustered acetylcholine receptors in the diagnosis of seronegative myasthenia gravis. *JAMA Neurol* **72:** 642–649.

Sanders DB, Siddiqi ZA (2008) Lessons from two trials of mycophenolate mofetil in myasthenia gravis. *Ann N Y Acad Sci* **1132:** 249–253.

Sanders DB, El-Salem K, Massey JM, McConville J, Vincent A (2003) Clinical aspects of MuSK antibody positive seronegative MG. *Neurology* **60:** 1978–1980.

Sanders DB, Hart IK, Mantegazza R et al. (2008) An international, phase III, randomized trial of mycophenolate mofetil in myasthenia gravis. *Neurology* **71:** 400–406.

Sanders DB, Wolfe GI, Benatar M et al. (2016) International consensus guidance for management of myasthenia gravis: executive summary. *Neurology* **87:** 419–425.

Sarrigiannis PG, Kennett RP, Read S, Farrugia ME (2006) Single-fiber EMG with a concentric needle electrode: validation in myasthenia gravis. *Muscle Nerve* **33:** 61–65.

Scuderi F, Marino M, Colonna L et al. (2002) Anti-p110 autoantibodies identify a subtype of 'seronegative' myasthenia gravis with prominent oculobulbar involvement. *Lab Invest* **82:** 1139–1146.

Selcen D, Dabrowski ER, Michon AM, Nigro MA (2000) High-dose intravenous immunoglobulin therapy in juvenile myasthenia gravis. *Pediatr Neurol* **22:** 40–43.

Seybold ME (1998) Thymectomy in childhood myasthenia gravis. *Ann N Y Acad Sci* **841:** 731–741.

Skeie GO, Apostolski S, Evoli A et al. (2006) Guidelines for the treatment of autoimmune neuromuscular transmission disorders. *Eur J Neurol* **13:** 691–699.

Sommer N, Melms A, Weller M, Dichgans J (1993) Ocular myasthenia gravis. A critical review of clinical and pathophysiological aspects. *Doc Ophthalmol* **84:** 309–333.

Sussman J, Farrugia ME, Maddison P, Hill M, Leite MI, Hilton-Jones D (2015) Myasthenia gravis: association of British Neurologists' management guidelines. *Pract Neurol* **15:** 199–206.

Tandan R, Hehir MK II, Waheed W, Howard DB (2017) Rituximab treatment of myasthenia gravis: A systematic review. *Muscle Nerve* **56:** 185–196.

Téllez-Zenteno JF, Hernández-Ronquillo L, Salinas V, Estanol B, da Silva O (2004) Myasthenia gravis and pregnancy: clinical implications and neonatal outcome. *BMC Musculoskelet Disord* **5:** 42.

Tracy MM, McRae W, Millichap JG (2009) Graded response to thymectomy in children with myasthenia gravis. *J Child Neurol* **24:** 454–459.

Tsonis AI, Zisimopoulou P, Lazaridis K et al. (2015) MuSK autoantibodies in myasthenia gravis detected by cell based assay – A multinational study. *J Neuroimmunol* **284:** 10–17.

Vernet-der Garabedian B, Lacokova M, Eymard B et al. (1994) Association of neonatal myasthenia gravis with antibodies against the fetal acetylcholine receptor. *J Clin Invest* **94:** 555–559.

Vincent A (2002) Unravelling the pathogenesis of myasthenia gravis. *Nat Rev Immunol* **2:** 797–804.

Vincent A, Newsom-Davis J (1985) Acetylcholine receptor antibody as a diagnostic test for myasthenia gravis: results in 153 validated cases and 2967 diagnostic assays. *J Neurol Neurosurg Psychiatry* **48:** 1246–1252.

Vincent A, Palace J, Hilton-Jones D (2001) Myasthenia gravis. *Lancet* **357:** 2122–2128.

Vincent A, Lang B, Kleopa KA (2006) Autoimmune channelopathies and related neurological disorders. *Neuron* **52:** 123–138.

Vincent A, Leite MI (2005) Neuromuscular junction autoimmune disease: muscle specific kinase antibodies and treatments for myasthenia gravis. *Curr Opin Neurol* **18:** 519–525.

Wolfe GI, Kaminski HJ, Aban IB et al. (2016) Randomized trial of thymectomy in myasthenia gravis. *N Engl J Med* **375:** 511–522.

Wong V, Hawkins BR, Yu YL (1992) Myasthenia gravis in Hong Kong Chinese. 2. Paediatric disease. *Acta Neurol Scand* **86:** 68–72.

Wylam ME, Anderson PM, Kuntz NL, Rodríguez V (2003) Successful treatment of refractory myasthenia gravis using rituximab: a pediatric case report. *J Pediatr* **143:** 674–677.

Zambelis T, Kokotis P, Karandreas N (2011) Repetitive nerve stimulation of facial and hypothenar muscles: relative sensitivity in different myasthenia gravis subgroups. *Eur Neurol* **65:** 203–207.

Zhang X, Yang M, Xu J et al. (2007) Clinical and serological study of myasthenia gravis in HuBei Province, China. *J Neurol Neurosurg Psychiatry* **78:** 386–390.

Zhang B, Tzartos JS, Belimezi M et al. (2012) Autoantibodies to lipoprotein-related protein 4 in patients with double-seronegative myasthenia gravis. *Arch Neurol* **69:** 445–451.

Zinman L, Bril V (2008) IVIG treatment for myasthenia gravis: effectiveness, limitations, and novel therapeutic strategies. *Ann N Y Acad Sci* **1132:** 264–270.

Zisimopoulou P, Evangelakou P, Tzartos J et al. (2014) A comprehensive analysis of the epidemiology and clinical characteristics of anti-LRP4 in myasthenia gravis. *J Autoimmun* **52:** 139–145.

Congenital Myasthenic Syndromes

Sandeep Jayawant, Pedro M Rodríguez Cruz, Jacqueline Palace and David Beeson

INTRODUCTION

The congenital myasthenic syndromes (CMS) are a heterogeneous group of disorders caused by mutations in a series of different genes that affect neuromuscular transmission (Beeson et al. 2005; Engel et al. 2015). Clinicians in the 1970s recognised congenital myasthenia as a distinct entity from autoimmune myasthenia based on the presentation from birth, early infancy or childhood, positive family history, absence of detectable antibodies against the acetylcholine receptor (AChR) and non-response to immunosuppression. Diagnosis was largely based on detailed ultrastructural and neurophysiologic studies of the neuromuscular junctions (NMJs) and motor endplates (Engel et al. 1979, 1981). In the last two decades, advances in genetic diagnosis such as next generation sequencing have helped identify several mutations causing structural and functional abnormalities that compromise neuromuscular transmission and the phenotypes associated with these mutations (Beeson 2016). Table 6.1 highlights the increasing array of genetic abnormalities identified recently in CMS.

EPIDEMIOLOGY

Congenital myasthenia is a rare disorder of childhood with a detected prevalence of 9.2 per million children under the age of 18. It is equally prevalent among girls and boys with *CHNRE*, *DOK7* and *RAPSN* as the most common mutations identified with respective prevalence figures of 3.4, 2.5 and 1.6 per million children for each (Parr et al. 2014). There was some variation in reported prevalence figures for different regions of England, Scotland and Wales. Over 350 kinships were identified in the Oxford Congenital Myasthenia Service which is a national service for the United Kingdom (Beeson 2012). Table 6.2 shows the relative prevalence of the various genetic subtypes in the Oxford cohort.

PATHOPHYSIOLOGY

Early studies in congenital myasthenia focussed on detailed ultrastructural analysis of the NMJ, the motor endplate and electrophysiological studies with endplate acetylcholine esterase deficiency (AChE), putative abnormalities of the acetylcholine (ACh) induced ion channel and putative defect of ACh re-synthesis or mobilisation being described (Engel et al. 1977, 1979). Figure 6.1 shows the chemical and electrical changes that occur at the NMJ to generate a motor action potential at the endplate.

The chemical transmission at the nerve muscle junction resulting in the generation of an action potential and muscle contraction has been covered in Chapters 1 and 2. We briefly re-iterate it here to help

Table 6.1   Congenital myasthenic syndromes subtypes and associated genes

Congenital myasthenic syndrome	Gene
Ubiquitously expressed proteins	
N-glycosylation pathway	
GFPT1	*GFPT1*
DPAGT1	*DPAGT1*
ALG2	*ALG2*
ALG14	*ALG14*
GMPPB	*GMPPB*
Propyl-oligopeptidase	
PREPL	*PREPL*
Proteins with defined function at the neuromuscular junction	
Presynaptic	
Choline acetyltransferase	*CHAT*
Synaptotagmin	*SYT2*
SNAP25B	*SNAP25B*
Synaptic	
Endplate AChE deficiency	*COLQ*
Laminin b2 deficiency	*LAMB2*
Agrin	*AGRN*
Collagen 13A1	*COL13A1*
Postsynaptic	
Primary acetylcholine receptor deficiency	*CHRNA1, CHRNB1, CHRND, CHRNE*
Escobar syndrome	*CHRNG*
Rapsyn	*RAPSN*
DOK7	*DOK7*
Slow-channel syndrome	*CHRNA1, CHRNB1, CHRND, CHRNE*
Fast-channel syndrome	*CHRNA1, CHRNB1, CHRND, CHRNE*
Low-conductance syndrome	*CHRNE*
MuSK	*MUSK*
Plectin deficiency	*PLEC1*
Na-channel myasthenia	*SCN4A*
LRP4	*LRP4*

Reproduced from Beeson (2016) with permission.

with the understanding of the mutations affecting this process. Choline acetyltransferase (ChAT) binds acetate and choline to produce ACh in the nerve terminal. It is generated in little packets or quanta and packaged into vesicles. These vesicles release the ACh into the synapse by endocytosis. Binding of the ACh molecules to the receptor opens a voltage-gated sodium channel for a short period of time causing a

Table 6.2   Kinships in the Oxford Congenital Myasthenia Service

Syndrome kinships	CMS syndrome	Number
AChR deficiency	CHRNE	146
AChR deficiency	RAPSN	73
CMS with proximal weakness	DOK7	68
Slow channel	CHRNA/B/D/E	25
Fast channel	CHRNA/D/E	15
AChE deficiency	COLQ	20
Presynaptic	ChAT	8

Numbers of the more common congenital myasthenic syndromes analysed in Oxford, classified by genetic screening and functional analysis of mutations. Adapted from Beeson (2012).

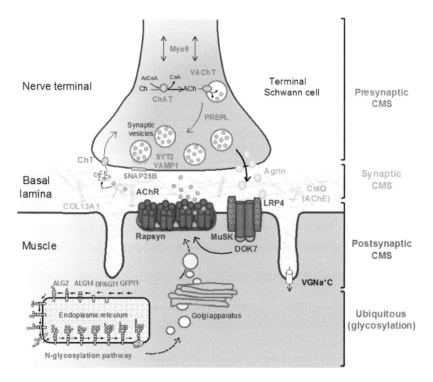

Figure 6.1   Schematic representation of the neuromuscular junction (NMJ) and the principle molecules involved in congenital myasthenia. The heterogeneous spectrum of mutated proteins and molecular mechanisms involved in congenital myasthenia syndromes (CMS) are illustrated. CMS results from presynaptic (ChAT, ChT, MUNC13-1, MYO9, PREPL, SYT2, VAChT, VAMP1), synaptic basal lamina abnormalities (COLQ, COL13A1) and postsynaptic defects (AChR subunits: α, β, δ and ε, AGRN, DOK7, MuSK, LRP4 and RAPSN). Additionally, the new genes encoding for molecules not confined to the NMJ (*GFPT1*, *DPAGT1*, *ALG2*, *ALG14* and *GMPPB*) are represented in the endoplasmic reticulum (ER), in a simplified view of the N-glycosylation pathway, together with the post-translational modifications of the saccharide structure of the AChR and other NMJ proteins inside the ER and Golgi apparatus, before reaching the muscle cell surface as mature proteins. ACh, acetylcholine; AChE, acetylcholinesterase; AcCoA, acetyl coenzyme A; AChR, acetylcholine receptor; Ch, choline; VGNa⁺C, voltage-gated sodium channel. Reproduced from Rodríguez Cruz et al. (2018) with permission. A colour version of this figure can be seen in the plate section.

depolarisation of the muscle fibre generating a miniature endplate potential (MEPP). Depolarisation of the nerve terminal opens a voltage sensitive calcium channel. The safety of neuromuscular transmission depends on exceeding the threshold required to generate an action potential. Acetylcholine then releases itself from the receptors and is hydrolysed by AChE into choline and acetate, the choline being taken up by the nerve terminal and utilised for re-synthesis of ACh (Engel 1988).

Based on the electrophysiological studies, CMS were classified into presynaptic, synaptic and postsynaptic disorders and the clinical criteria and laboratory criteria were established to make a diagnosis of these (Engel 1994; Middleton 1996). This classification remains in use to date even with better understanding of the genetics and pathophysiology of the newly identified CMS with further addition of the newly identified ubiquitously expressed proteins (Chaouch et al. 2012; Beeson 2016).

In this chapter we use the new genetic classification of CMS. Identification of distinct phenotypes can help direct the sequence of genetic investigation, although new generation sequencing will probably be the main diagnostic tool of the future.

CLINICAL PHENOTYPES OF CONGENITAL MYASTHENIC SYNDROMES

Presynaptic Abnormalities

CHOLINE ACETYL TRANSFERASE MUTATION

An autosomal recessive loss of function mutation impairs the synthesis of ACh in the nerve terminal. This rare CMS was first described by Ohno et al. in 2001 as a congenital myasthenia associated with episodic apnoeas. Mutation in the ChAT gene affects the catalytic activity of the transferase enzyme, expression levels of the enzyme or a combination of the two (Arredondo et al. 2015). This results in reduced filling of ACh molecules in the vesicles thus resulting in a reduced quantal release of ACh in the synaptic cleft (Beeson 2016). The vesicular acetylcholine transporter (VAChT) also acts to package the acetylcholine into vesicles. The VAChT gene is located within one of the introns of the ChAT gene. The ChAT gene also encodes for the VAChT; thus mutations in the ChAT that affect both the transferase enzyme and the transporter result in presynaptic dysfunction with reduced quantal release of acetylcholine in the synapse (Eiden 1998). Ohno et al. (2001) reported several kinships with ChAT mutations which were shown to reduce the expression and/or catalytic efficiency of ChAT. Characteristic clinical features reported were sudden episodes of severe dyspnoea and bulbar weakness leading to apnoea precipitated by infections, fever, excitement and unrelated stressors such as other diseases or drugs that affect neuromuscular transmission. Some patients presented at birth with hypotonia and severe bulbar and respiratory weakness requiring ventilatory support that slowly improved with time, but episodes of apnoea and bulbar paralysis recurred later in life. Other patients first experienced attacks during infancy or early childhood. Variable ptosis and muscle weakness persisted between the attacks. Crises may be prevented or mitigated by use of anticholinesterase drugs. A decremental electromyogram (EMG) response was absent in rested muscles but could be elicited after a conditioning train of 10Hz stimuli for 5 minutes. After stimulation, the decreased compound muscle action potential (CMAP) amplitude recovered slowly over several minutes (Ohno et al. 2001; Schmidt et al. 2003). In between crisis episodes the signs and symptoms may be very mild with little evidence of ptosis, normal eye movements and minimal skeletal muscle fatigue. Treatment is with AChE inhibitors or 3,4-diaminopyridine (DAP). This should be considered in the diagnosis where there is a family history of sudden unexpected deaths especially in infancy (Byring et al. 2002). The crisis gets less frequent after the first decade of life.

Other Rare Presynaptic Congenital Myasthenic Syndromes

Some rare mutations in various genes also affect presynaptic transmission.

SLC5A7/CHT MUTATION

Recessive mutations in the *SLC5A7* gene cause a severe form of presynaptic CMS affecting brain development and cognition. It affects function of the hemicholinium-3 sensitive choline transporter (CHT/SLC5A7) which is responsible for re-uptake of choline after ACh is cleaved into choline and acetate by the action of AChE. Reported clinical phenotype is of generalised hypotonia, respiratory insufficiency, apnoea, bulbar and extra ocular muscle involvement, generalised fatigable weakness and decrement on repetitive nerve stimulation (Pardal-Fernández et al. 2018). Treatment is with AChE inhibitors.

SYNAPTOTAGMIN (SYT2) MUTATION

This mutation is predicted to produce a conformational change in the C2B domain of synaptotagmin that would decrease Ca^{2+} binding. When expressed in Drosophila containing no synaptotagmin, this mutation was lethal, demonstrating the critical nature of the examined residue. When expressed in combination with wild-type synaptotagmin, it results in decreased Ca^{2+} affinity for neurotransmitter release and a decreased release probability (Shields et al. 2017). This mutation results in a presynaptic CMS with motor neuropathy causing lower limb wasting, foot deformity, reflex potentiation following exercise, a uniquely prolonged post-tetanic potentiation period on neurophysiology and response to treatment with AChE inhibitors and 3,4-DAP (Herrmann et al. 2014; Whittaker et al. 2015).

Synaptosomal-associated protein mutation (*SNAP25*) cause a phenotype of myasthenia, ataxia, epilepsy and intellectual disability (Shen et al. 2014).

SYNAPTOBREVIN

Synaptobrevin (SYB1)/VAMP1 is one of the three core SNARE (soluble N-ethylmaleimide-sensitive factor attachment protein receptor) components of the synaptic vesicle fusion machinery. Synaptobrevin 1 attached to the synaptic vesicles is a v-SNARE; syntaxin and SNAP25B anchored in the target presynaptic membrane are t-SNAREs (Sudhoff et al. 2017; Shen et al. 2017). The reported case by Shen et al. presented at birth with severe weakness, hypotonia, limited ocular ductions, and bulbar symptoms. Cases reported with *VAMP1* mutations showed arthrogryposis, delayed motor development, feeding difficulties, strabismus, ophthalmoplegia and respiratory difficulties with frequent respiratory infections (Salpietro et al. 2017) The initial low amplitude of single evoked muscle action potentials and their marked potentiation by high frequency nerve stimulation (see Fig. 6.1 B and D) pointed to a presynaptic defect. The patient sadly passed away from respiratory failure after an infection at age 14 (Shen et al. 2017).

MYOSIN ENCODING GENE

Loss of myosin encoding gene (MYO9A) affects the neuronal cytoskeleton and leads to impaired transport of proteins, including agrin. The phenotype is of a severe neonatal presentation with respiratory and bulbar involvement, swallowing difficulties, proximal and distal muscle weakness, delayed motor milestones, episodic apnoea, ophthalmoplegia, nystagmus ptosis (O'Connor et al. 2016, 2018). There was good response to treatment with pyridostigmine and 3,4-DAP.

PROLYL ENDOPEPTIDASE-LIKE GENE MUTATIONS

Prolyl endopeptidase-like gene mutations (*PREPL*) can occur with or without cystinuria. The hypotonia-cystinuria syndrome (HCS) is characterised by cystinuria in combination with severe neonatal hypotonia, fluctuating ptosis, facial paresis, dysarthria and feeding problems suggesting a myasthenic disorder and growth hormone deficiency. Other features are viscous saliva and hypergonadotrophic hypogonadism, and half of the patients need special education The hypotonia and feeding problems improve during the first year of life, but ptosis, nasal voice, dysarthria, facial weakness and mild axial and proximal muscle weakness persist. Hyperphagia with tendency to obesity develops during childhood. HCS is caused by autosomal recessive deletions involving two contiguous genes on chromosome 2p21: *SLC3A1*, which encodes the heavy subunit of the cysteine dibasic and neutral amino acid transporter (OMIM 104614), and *PREPL*, the prolyl endopeptidase-like gene (Régal et al. 2014).

SLC18A3 MUTATIONS

Mutations in *SLC18A3* result in a severe autosomal recessive congenital myasthenic syndrome affecting function of the vesicular ACh transporter. It is characterised by severe hypotonia, arthrogryposis and respiratory failure (Aran et al. 2017). Chromosomal deletions in 10q11.2 associated with *ChAT* or *SLC18A3* have been described (Schwartz et al. 2018). Reported cases presented with hypotonia, sleep apnoea, chronic constipation, gastro-oesophageal reflux, nystagmus and ptosis.

LAMININ MUTATION

There are isolated case reports of patients with laminin (LAMA5) mutation resulting in a presynaptic deficit of neuromuscular transmission. It involves both reduction of the pool of synaptic vesicles readily available for release and a diminished probability of vesicle release, similar to that seen in Lambert–Eaton myasthenic syndrome. There is good response to a combined treatment with pyridostigmine and 3,4-DAP. The patient reported had ptosis, high arched palate, respiratory distress requiring tracheostomy but no apnoeas, hypotonia, proximal weakness and neck flexion weakness (Maselli et al. 2018).

MAMMALIAN UNCO-ORDINATED PROTEIN

Very few patients with mammlian unco-ordinated protein (MUNC13-1) have been identified. The reported patient had severe myasthenic symptoms at birth with poor spontaneous movements, variable ptosis, high arched palate, small jaw, kyphoscoliosis, clinodactyly and contractures of proximal joints and knees. The electroencephalogram showed sharp waves without clinical seizures. EMG showed decrement and abnormalities similar to Lambert–Eaton syndrome, characterising it as a presynaptic defect with increased CMAP amplitude on nerve stimulation at 50Hz. Treatment with pyridostigmine and 3,4-DAP improved the patients cry and cough but did not improve limb power. She died at 50 months age of respiratory failure following a chest infection. MUNC13 associates with SNAP25B and synaptobrevin to form primed SNARE complexes thereby preparing synaptic vesicles for exocytosis (Ma et al. 2013; Engel et al. 2018). It is inherited in an autosomal recessive pattern.

Synaptic Abnormalities

COLLAGEN TAIL MUTATION

Collagen tail (*COLQ*) mutation causes a defect in the collagen tail of the enzyme AChE. Absence of AChE prolongs the time ACh remains in the synaptic cleft. This in turn increases the duration of the endplate current so that it outlasts the refractory period of the muscle fibre and excites a second CMAP. The prolonged endplate currents lead to overload of the synaptic space with cations and cause an endplate myopathy with loss of acetylcholine receptors. Electron microscopy studies of endplates of patients with *COLQ* mutations revealed degeneration of the junctional folds and abnormally small nerve terminals encased by Schwann cells (Engel et al. 2003). Collagen tail (*COLQ*) mutation is characterised by onset during childhood, generalised weakness increased by exertion, refractoriness to anticholinesterase drugs, decremental electromyographic response and morphological abnormalities of the NMJs (Engel et al. 1977). The disease often manifests at birth. Muscle hypotonia, ptosis, ophthalmoparesis, poor head control, poor cry and suck, respiratory insufficiency are the presenting symptoms in the neonatal period (Mihaylova et al. 2008). Respiratory crises occur through early childhood and may be lethal. Proximal weakness with waddling gait and an internal rotation of the knees with crossing of the legs is often seen. Slow pupillary response to light is an inconsistent finding. Double CMAP response on repetitive nerve stimulation with increased jitter on single fibre EMG (SFEMG) may be seen. Although there may be some short term response to AChE inhibitors, there is either no sustained improvement or worsening on continued use of AChE inhibitors. Patients often respond to ephedrine or salbutamol (Albuterol) although the response may not be evident for several weeks and may continue for many months after treatment initiation.

LAMININ BETA 2 MUTATION

Laminin beta 2 (*LAMB2*) mutation causes a rare form of congenital myasthenia with neonatal respiratory distress, constricted pupils and a microcystic nephropathy. There is worsening of the weakness with cholinesterase inhibitors. Ocular findings include miosis, ptosis, ophthalmoplegia, decreased visual acuity with hypoplastic macula. In the patient reported there was decreased average axon terminal area and reduced numbers of synaptic vesicles per area. The width of the synaptic cleft was increased and there was reduction of the endplate index. This results from single base pair deletions leading to frame shifts and thereby truncated proteins. This results in failure of assembly of the laminin subunits. It is inherited in an autosomal recessive pattern. Treatment with 3,4-DAP may be beneficial. Renal transplantation may increase survival rates and longevity (Maselli et al. 2009).

COLLAGEN 13 ALPHA

Mutations in collagen 13 alpha (*COL13A1*) cause a synaptic neuromuscular transmission defect. It encodes an extracellular matrix protein that is concentrated in the NMJ. This is required for maintaining synaptic stability. It is inherited in an autosomal recessive pattern. Symptoms are evident in the neonatal period with respiratory and feeding difficulties, mild facial dysmorphism, ptosis but normal eye movements, and marked weakness of neck flexion. Children may also show pectus carinatum chest deformity. Ptosis may become fixed over time and there may be some improvement in the myasthenic weakness over time. There is no response to cholinesterase inhibitors but patients reported improvement on salbutamol and 3,4-DAP (Beeson et al. 2018).

AGRIN

Agrin (AGRN) encodes an extracellular matrix proteoglycan involved in the development and maintenance of the NMJ. This proteoglycan is a key organiser of the postsynaptic membrane through stabilisation and maintenance of postsynaptic acetylcholine receptors (AChRs) formed on muscle fibres (McMahan et al. 1992). A neural isoform of agrin is secreted from the nerve terminal into the synaptic basement membrane and binds a postsynaptic transmembrane receptor (low-density lipoprotein receptor-related protein 4; LRP4), which activates the muscle-specific kinase (MuSK) to induce the stabilisation of AChR clusters and the establishment of new clusters (Kim et al. 2008). Autosomal recessive missense mutations in the *AGRN* gene were shown to lead to congenital myasthenic syndrome characterised by ptosis and global fatigable limb weakness and some with distal myopathy features with neurophysiological evidence of neuromuscular transmission defect (Nicole et al. 2014).

Postsynaptic Abnormalities

These are the commonest congenital myasthenias. The nicotinic AChR of skeletal muscle is a neurotransmitter-gated ion channel composed of five subunits that mediates synaptic transmission at the vertebrate NMJ. Mutations in its subunit genes cause postsynaptic CMS. AChR deficiency syndromes thus arise from either AChR subunit (mainly epsilon subunit) mutations or receptor associated protein at the synapse (RAPSN) mutations, each with distinct phenotypes. Mutations of the AChR subunits can also lead to abnormal kinetic function of the receptor leading to the slow- and fast-channel syndromes (Palace and Beeson 2008). Mutations in the gamma AChR subunit (fetal form) cause fetal akinesia and has recently been recognised as a cause of severe arthrogryposis and multiple pterigium associated with Escobar syndrome in neonates (Hoffmann et al. 2006). However, because the adult (epsilon) subunit replaces the gamma in utero, childhood muscle weakness is not a feature. Other mutations in the alpha and delta subunits and in RAPSN cause fetal akinesia deformation sequence disorders (Michalk et al. 2008). *DOK7* mutations lead to a NMJ synaptopathy. Additionally, there are two single case reports of CMS due to respective heteroallelic mutations in the postsynaptic sodium channel (*SCN4A*) and in MuSK (Tsujino et al. 2003; Chevessier et al. 2004). Other mutations in *AGRN* and *LRP4* cause defects in endplate development and maintenance. Recently, defects in protein glycosylation have been identified (*GFPT1*, *DPAGT1*, *ALG2*, *ALG14*, *GMPPB*) leading to CMS. The muscle AChR is a glycoprotein with all subunits known to undergo N-linked glycosylation. Glycosylation is an essential process in the assembly and transport of the AChR into the postsynaptic membrane, these mutations therefore result in reduced endplate AChR number (Ohno 2013).

ACETYLCHOLINE RECEPTOR DEFICIENCY

CMS with endplate AChR deficiency result from different homozygous or heterozygous recessive mutations in genes encoding the various subunits of the AChR (α, β, δ and ε). The most common subunit mutation is the epsilon subunit. This is probably because the fetal gamma subunit, which is replaced in utero by the epsilon subunit, by expressing itself at low levels affords some protection in epsilon mutation patients whereas those harbouring non-epsilon null mutations may not survive because of the severe phenotype. Also, the gene encoding the epsilon subunit, and especially exons coding for the long cytoplasmic loop, has a high guanosine-cytosine content that likely predisposes to DNA rearrangements (Beeson et al. 2005).

EPSILON MUTATION CONGENTIAL MYASTHENIC SYNDROMES

Children with epsilon subunit mutations present with ptosis and ophthalmoplegia within infancy. Other features are bulbar and facial weakness as well as generalised skeletal weakness (Croxen et al. 1998). They show a mild clinical phenotype with exacerbations during inter current illness. They rarely deteriorate much over time and show a very good clinical response to AChE inhibitors. It is important to note that ptosis may respond to pyridostigmine and 3,4-DAP but the ophthalmoplegia rarely improves on treatment. Inheritance is autosomal recessive. Other mutations in the epsilon subunit can also cause kinetic abnormalities of the AChR resulting in prolonged openings and an endplate myopathy (Ohno et al. 1995).

OTHER SUBUNIT MUTATIONS CAUSING ACETYLCHOLINE RECEPTOR DEFICIENCY

Mutations of other receptors also cause a deficiency of available AChRs resulting in impaired neuromuscular transmission. Other mechanisms, such as clustering of the receptors, effect on channel opening times etc., may also play a role (Shen et al. 2002; Müller et al. 2006).

Kinetic abnormalities of the acetylcholine receptor

Mutations in the other AChR subunit genes – ε, α, β and δ – can also cause abnormal opening and closing of the AChR channels. These are voltage-gated sodium channels which by patch clamp electrophysiologic studies have shown prolonged channel burst duration or abbreviated burst duration (Beeson 2012) (Fig. 6.2).

Slow-channel syndrome

The slow-channel congenital myasthenic syndrome was first described in 1982 (Engel et al. 1982). It is one of the only autosomal dominant forms of CMS apart from SYT2, and is due to mutations within the AChR subunits that cause prolonged activation of the AChR ion channel (Ohno et al. 1995; Sine et al. 1995). Weakness of cervical, scapular and finger extensor muscles is often an early feature. The disorder is commonly slowly progressive affecting respiratory, limb and bulbar muscles (Engel 2015). Symptoms may be present at birth or may not develop until well into adulthood. Severity can vary from mild to severe, although it tends to be slowly progressive. Diagnostic features include selective weakness of cervical, scapular, and finger extensor muscles, an absent response to anticholinesterase medication, and a double response to a single nerve stimulus during electromyography, which is common but not invariable (Croxen et al. 2002). Patients do not respond to ACh and may deteriorate. It responds to long-acting

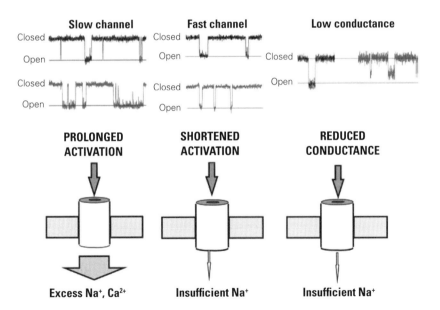

Figure 6.2   Illustration of the pathogenic mechanisms of disorders of the acetylcholine receptor ion channel. Top panels illustrate patch clamp single acetylcholine receptor channel recording traces: black traces, wild-type channels; red traces, mutant channels. Lower panels illustrate the consequence of altered ion channel function. Reproduced from Beeson (2012) with permission from Wiley. A colour version of this figure can be seen in the plate section.

open channel blocking agents, fluoxetine or quinidine. Treatment should be carefully monitored as both fluoxetine can have significant side effects with suicidal ideation and cardiac arrhythmias with quinidine (Colomer et al. 2006). Serum drug levels for both can be used for monitoring.

FAST-CHANNEL SYNDROME

Autosomal recessive mutations in the alpha, delta and epsilon subunits can cause a shortened activation of the AChR channel resulting in a fast-channel syndrome. Patients present at birth with respiratory and/ or bulbar problems and congenital stridor, ptosis and ophthalmoplegia, and neck, jaw and facial weakness as well as proximal limb muscle weakness. Mild contractures may be seen. Abrupt life threatening acute respiratory crises and apnoeic attacks can be severe in infancy but ease after childhood. They show a partial response to cholinesterase inhibitors and 3,4-DAP (Palace et al. 2012). They show good response to pyridostigmine and 3,4-DAP. Parental training in the emergency use of non-invasive ventilator support may be helpful (Robb et al. 2010).

SCN4A (SODIUM CHANNEL MUTATION)

Rare cases of autosomal recessive sodium channel mutations have been described in patients with features of congenital myasthenia with periodic paralysis. They may respond to pyridostigmine and acetazolamide. Abrupt attacks of respiratory and bulbar paralysis from birth, delayed motor development, hypotonia ptosis, ophthalmoplegia, high arched palate and non-painful muscle contractions precipitated by cold have been described. No myotonic discharges were detected on electromyograms (Tsujino et al. 2003; Habbout et al. 2016).

RECEPTOR ASSOCIATED PROTEIN AT THE SYNAPSE (RAPSN)

This is one of the commonest CMS. Rapsyn forms part of a "core pathway" that is responsible for initiating and maintaining the specialised postsynaptic structures at the NMJ (Burke et al. 2003). Rapsyn N88K, has been found as a frequent cause of congenital myasthenic syndrome originating from central or western Europe (Müller et al. 2003). Mutations in this gene result in two distinct phenotypes – early and late onset. Early-onset phenotypes present with arthrogryposis multiplex congenita at birth with jaw and palate deformities, strabismus but not ophthalmoplegia, respiratory failure and episodic crises. They also improve later in life, and despite the severe symptoms at birth, the majority experience little disability in the long run. The respiratory crises reduce in frequency and intensity through school years and are rarely seen in adult age. They respond very well to cholinesterase inhibitors. The late-onset phenotype patients have ankle dorsiflexion weakness as a characteristic feature. Weakness and wasting of distal upper limb muscles is also seen. They do not respond very well to cholinesterase inhibitors. They need to be considered in the differential diagnosis of seronegative myasthenia gravis patients (Burke et al. 2003).

DOWNSTREAM OF KINASE 7

Downstream of kinase 7 (DOK7) is a member of the DOK-family of proteins, which are adaptor molecules that act as downstream activators of receptor tyrosine kinases (Okada et al. 2006). This congenital myasthenic syndrome, which is one of the more common subtypes was first described in 2006 (Beeson et al. 2006). Recessive mutations in this gene cause fatigable weakness in a limb-girdle distribution (Cossins et al. 2012). It can however present from birth with bulbar weakness, hypotonia and ptosis. Apnoea, contractures, ophthalmoplegia and strabismus are rarely seen and walking is not usually significantly delayed. Waddling and lordotic gait resulting from proximal lower limb weakness is seen. Shoulder girdle weakness soon follows. Facial, jaw and neck weakness is often seen with tongue wasting (Palace et al.

2007). There is a reduction in postsynaptic endplate area which could limit the effectiveness of increasing endplate ACh with pyridostigmine and increase the risk of depolarisation blockade (Slater et al. 2006). This is probably why DOK7 patients do not respond well to pyridostigmine or get worse. They improve with 3,4-DAP or ephedrine which probably works by increasing quantal release of ACh (Sieb and Engel 1993). Both Salbutamol and Ephedrine work over a longer period of time by repairing synaptic structure.

LOW-DENSITY LIPOPROTEIN RECEPTOR-RELATED PROTEIN MUTATION

Low-density lipoprotein receptor-related protein (LRP4) is a transmembrane protein of the postsynaptic membrane. LRP binds to agrin and forms a ternary complex with the postsynaptic transmembrane muscle-specific tyrosine kinase (MuSK). In this complex, the third β-propeller domain of LRP4 is important for association with MuSK. Recessive mutations in this gene cause a congenital myasthenic syndrome characterised by respiratory distress and apnoea from birth, ptosis, ophthalmoplegia, delayed motor milestones and progressive proximal weakness which may result in loss of independent ambulation. They may get worse on treatment with pyridostigmine and 3,4-DAP, but may respond to longer term treatment with salbutamol/albuterol (Ohkawara et al. 2014; Selcen et al. 2015).

PLEC1 (PLECTIN)

Plectin, a 466 kD cytoskeleton linker protein encoded by the *PLEC1* gene on 8q24, is expressed abundantly in epithelia and muscle with an important role in maintaining cytoarchitectural integrity. A rare form of muscular dystrophy with early-onset blistering skin condition epidermolysis bullosa has been described with neuromuscular transmission defect. The described patient responded to 3,4-DAP but not pyridostigmine. Other patients reported have ptosis, fatigable weakness and extraocular muscle weakness (Forrest et al. 2010).

MUSCLE-SPECIFIC KINASE

Missense mutations in the gene encoding muscle-specific kinase (MuSK) cause a postsynaptic congenital myasthenic syndrome with a severe phenotype. Neural agrin activates MuSK which plays a role in clustering of AChRs. Cases reported have weakness and respiratory difficulties with onset at birth or during infancy; no delay of initial motor milestones; and, a pattern of proximal limb-girdle weakness, which does not associate with significant impairment of external ocular movements. There is little response to pyridostigmine or 3,4-DAP but patients improve with salbutamol/albuterol (Maselli et al. 2010).

Ubiquitous Defects

GLYCOSYLATION DISORDERS

Mutations in five additional genes have been reported as causing limb-girdle phenotype CMS (LG-CMS). They encode for ubiquitous proteins involved in the glycosylation pathway: *GFPT1* (glutamine-fructose-6-phosphate transaminase 1), *DPAGT1* (dolichyl-phosphate *N*-acetylglucosamine phosphotransferase 1), *ALG2* (alpha-1,3-mannosyltransferase), *ALG14* (UDP-*N*-acetylglucosaminyltransferase subunit) and most recently *GMPPB* (GDP-mannose pyrophosphorylase B) (Fig. 6.3).

Glutamine-fructose 6 phosphate transaminase 1

Mutations in this gene, encoding an enzyme involved in glycosylation of ubiquitous proteins, cause a limb-girdle congenital myasthenic syndrome (LG-CMS) with tubular aggregates (TAs) characterised predominantly by affection of the proximal skeletal muscles and presence of highly organised and remodelled

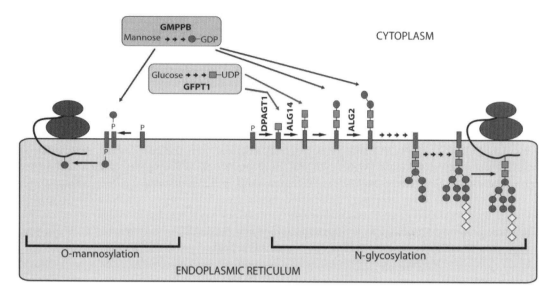

Figure 6.3   Simplified scheme of N-linked and O-linked glycosylation showing the five glycosylation genes (*GFPT1*, *DPAGT1*, *ALG2*, *ALG14* and *GMPPB*) associated with the congenital myasthenia syndromes. Reproduced from Belaya et al. (2015) with permission from Oxford University Press. A colour version of this figure can be seen in the plate section.

sarcoplasmic tubules in patients' muscle biopsies (Bauché et al. 2017). GFPTs are homodimeric, cytoplasmic enzymes that transfer an amino group from glutamine onto fructose-6-phosphate yielding glucosamine-6-phosphate (GlcN-6-P) and glutamate. This reaction is the first and rate-limiting step of the hexosamine biosynthesis pathway, which is the obligatory source of essential building blocks used for the synthesis of glycoproteins, glycolipids, and proteoglycans. Many key NMJ proteins are glycosylated, including MuSK, AChR subunits, agrin, dystroglycan, and integrins. Mutations result in reduced AChR numbers at the endplate shown in Zebrafish model studies (Senderek et al. 2011). It is inherited in an autosomal recessive pattern. Clinical features include fatigable proximal muscle weakness from early childhood, involving shoulder and pelvic girdle, wrist extensors, with progressive weakness resulting in loss of ambulation. There is relative sparing of facial, ocular and respiratory muscles. There is good response to pyridostigmine and 3,4-DAP (Zoltowska et al. 2013).

Dolichyl-phosphate N-acetylglucosamine phosphotransferase 1

This is another protein involved in the N-glycosylation pathway which when mutated impairs function of one of the NMJ. This endoplasmic reticulum-resident transmembrane protein catalyses the transfer of N-acetylglucosamine from cytosolic UDP-N-acetylglucosamine to dolichol-phosphate, which is also located in the endoplasmic reticulum membrane. The result is the formation of dolichol-pyrophosphate-N-acetylglucosamine, the carrier of the sugars that are finally attached to proteins in glycosylation (Yuste-Checa et al. 2017). The end result is a loss of endplate AChR. It is inherited in an autosomal recessive pattern. Muscle biopsies in those affected show tubular aggregates as with GFPT1 and the clinical phenotype is very similar with proximal limb-girdle distribution weakness and some wrist extension weakness but with minimal involvement of ocular, facial and bulbar muscles with onset in later childhood. There is good response to pyridostigmine and 3,4-DAP (Belaya et al. 2012).

Asparagine-linked glycosylation proteins

ALG14 is thought to form a multi-glycosyltransferase complex with ALG13 and DPAGT1 that catalyses the first two committed steps of asparagine-linked protein glycosylation. ALG14 is concentrated at the muscle motor endplates and mutations result in reduced cell-surface expression of muscle acetylcholine receptor. ALG2 is an alpha-1, 3-mannosyltransferase that also catalyses early steps in the asparagine-linked glycosylation pathway. It is inherited in an autosomal recessive pattern. Clinical features include fatigable proximal weakness, mild facial weakness but no bulbar or ocular involvement. There may be proximal joint contractures with a high arched palate. The condition remains stable through adult life after presentation in early childhood with delayed motor milestones, frequent falls and waddling gait and some never achieve independent ambulation. Muscle biopsy shows non-specific myopathic features, sometimes with tubular aggregates in older patients. There is good response to pyridostigmine and 3,4-DAP (Cossins et al. 2013).

Guanosine diphosphate mannose pyrophosphorylase B

A spectrum of clinical phenotypes associated with GMPPB mutations that stretched from defective neuromuscular transmission forming the major symptomatic component to GMPPB-MDDG cases with a limb-girdle muscular dystrophy in which no detectable NMJ defect have been identified (Belaya et al. 2015). Clinical features consist of variable weakness of proximal limb muscle groups with sparing of facial and eye muscles. However, patients with GMPPB–CMS had more prominent myopathic features that were detectable on muscle biopsies, electromyography, muscle magnetic resonance imaging, and through elevated serum creatine kinase levels. A dystroglycanopathy has been described with GMPPB mutations. It is inherited in an autosomal recessive pattern with presentation in childhood or adolescence. Muscle biopsy may show dystrophic features with reduced staining with alpha dystroglycan. Patients have shown some response to pyridostigmine (Belaya et al. 2015; Luo et al. 2017).

FETAL HYPOKINESIA AND ARTHROGRYPOSIS MULTIPLEX CONGENITA

Fetal hypokinesia can be caused by many neuromuscular conditions including congenital myasthenia. Mutations in many of the CMS genes including *RAPSN* and AChR subunits can cause fetal akinesia and contractures at birth. Escobar or multiple pterygia syndrome, a form of arthrogryposis multiplex congenita, is an autosomal recessive condition characterised by excessive webbing (pterygia), congenital contractures (arthrogryposis),and scoliosis. Other features include intrauterine death, congenital respiratory distress, short stature, facio-cranial dysmorphism, ptosis, low set ears, arachnodactyly and cryptorchidism in males. Several families with Escobar syndrome are found to have a mutation in the fetal gamma subunit of the AChR. As the gamma subunit is not expressed after birth these children have contractures but no myasthenic symptoms. Scoliosis, arachnodactyly, high arched palates, facial weakness and respiratory distress are some of the clinical features (Hoffmann et al. 2006).

MUSCLE DISORDERS WITH NEUROMUSCULAR TRANSMISSION DEFECTS

Several muscle disorders have been shown to have neuromuscular transmission defects. Some will partially respond to treatment with cholinesterase inhibitors improving power and function. They are covered elsewhere in this book.

DIAGNOSIS OF CONGENITAL MYASTHENIC SYNDROMES

Diagnosis of CMS rests on a high index of suspicion. Some historical features and clinical features that should alert a physician to the diagnosis are listed in Table 6.3.

It is very important to elicit a history suggestive of muscle fatigue. Examples of this are ptosis that is more evident towards the end of the day, volume of speech that gets weaker, fatigue of hand muscles after writing for some time, difficulty with stairs, difficulty getting up from sitting, suck that gets weak with time thus taking a long time to feed and choking with feeds, chewing or swallowing difficulties, running awkwardly and slower than peers in school. Recurrent episodes of chest infections with wheeze or stridor often labelled as "recurrent bronchiolitis" should raise suspicion. Apnoeic episodes and family history of sudden infant deaths should be investigated carefully.

Once there is a clinical suspicion of CMS, electrophysiology provides supportive evidence. Single fibre EMG demonstrating increased jitter is a very sensitive tool but technically difficult to achieve. Modified techniques such as stimulated EMG potential analysis using concentric electrodes (SPACE) to evaluate NMJ disorders in awake children have been developed (Pitt et al. 2017). This technique uses high frequency filtration of stimulated motor unit potentials and applies peak detection software to estimate mean consecutive difference (MCD). This has been covered extensively in Chapter 2.

The most widely used genetic tools were PCR-based studies of exons, exon–intron junctions and promoter regions of CMS genes, by direct sequencing. This classic approach detects point mutations and small insertions/deletions and is integrated in a sequential testing of gene-after-gene strategy, depending on clinical and EMG data (Chaouch et al. 2012). Re-sequencing microarrays can help detect missense mutations but may miss insertions and deletions (Denning et al. 2007). Targeted next generation sequencing (NGS) can be very useful for rapid testing using a panel of known CMS genes or for identifying new candidate genes in hitherto undiagnosed cases (Das et al. 2014).

Table 6.3   Historical and clinical features suggestive of a diagnosis of congenital myasthenic syndromes

Fetal bradykinesia and fetal distress

Polyhydramnios

Feeding difficulties

Weak suck and swallow

Weak cry

Arthrogryposis

Facial weakness

Ptosis

Strabismus and ophthalmoplegia

High arched palate

Proximal skeletal muscle weakness

Distal muscle weakness

Delayed motor milestones

Stridor

Recurrent chest infections and apnoeic episodes

Recurrent choking episodes

Scoliosis

REFERENCES

Aran A, Segel R, Kaneshige K et al. (2017) Vesicular acetylcholine transporter defect underlies devastating congenital myasthenia syndrome. *Neurology* **88:** 1021–1028.

Arredondo J, Lara M, Gospe SM Jr et al. (2015) Choline acetyltransferase mutations causing congenital myasthenic syndromes: molecular findings and genotype–phenotype correlations. *Hum Mutat* **36:** 881–893.

Bauché S, Vellieux G, Sternberg D et al. (2017) Mutations in GFPT1-related congenital myasthenic syndromes are associated with synaptic morphological defects and underlie a tubular aggregate myopathy with synaptopathy. *J Neurol* **264:** 1791–1803.

Beeson D (2012) Synaptic dysfunction in congenital myasthenic syndromes. *Ann N Y Acad Sci* **1275:** 63–69.

Beeson D (2016) Congenital myasthenic syndromes: recent advances. *Curr Opin Neurol* **29:** 565–571. https://journals.lww.com/co-neurology/pages/default.aspx

Beeson D, Hantaï D, Lochmüller H, Engel AG (2005) 126th International Workshop: Congenital Myasthenic Syndromes, 24–26 September 2004, Naarden, the Netherlands. *Neuromuscul Disord* **15:** 498–512.

Beeson D, Higuchi O, Palace J et al. (2006) Dok-7 mutations underlie a NMJ synaptopathy. *Science* **313:** 1975–1978.

Beeson D, Cossins J, Rodríguez-Cruz P, Maxwell S, Liu WW, Palace J (2018) Myasthenic syndromes due to defects in COL13A1 and in the N-linked glycosylation pathway. *Ann N Y Acad Sci* **1413:** 163–169.

Belaya K, Finlayson S, Slater CR et al. (2012) Mutations in DPAGT1 cause a limb-girdle congenital myasthenic syndrome with tubular aggregates. *Am J Hum Genet* **91:** 193–201.

Belaya K, Rodríguez Cruz P, Liu W et al. (2015). Mutations in GMPPB cause congenital myasthenic syndrome and bridge myasthenic disorders with dystroglycanopathies. *Brain* **138(9):** 2493–2504.

Burke G, Cossins J, Maxwell S et al. (2003) Rapsyn mutations in hereditary myasthenia: distinct early- and late-onset phenotypes. *Neurology* **61:** 826–828.

Byring RF, Pihko H, Tsujino A et al. (2002) Congenital myasthenic syndrome associated with episodic apnea and sudden infant death. *Neuromuscul Disord* **12:** 548–553.

Chaouch A, Beeson D, Hantaï D, Lochmüller H (2012) 186th ENMC International Workshop: Congenital Myasthenic Syndromes, 24–26 June 2011, Naarden, The Netherlands. *Neuromuscul Disord* **22:** 566–576.

Chevessier F, Faraut B, Ravel-Chapuis A et al. (2004) MuSK, a new target for mutations causing congenital myasthenic syndrome. *Hum Mol Genet* **13:** 3229–3240.

Colomer J, Müller JS, Vernet A et al. (2006) Long-term improvement of slow-channel congenital myasthenic syndrome with fluoxetine. *Neuromuscul Disord* **16:** 329–333.

Cossins J, Liu WW, Belaya K et al. (2012) The spectrum of mutations that underlie the neuromuscular junction synaptopathy in DOK7 congenital myasthenic syndrome. *Hum Mol Genet* **21:** 3765–3775.

Cossins J, Belaya K, Hicks D et al. (2012) Congenital myasthenic syndromes due to mutations in ALG2 and ALG14. *Brain* **136:** 944–956.

Croxen R, Beeson D, Newland C, Betty M, Vincent A, Newsom-Davis J (1998) A single nucleotide deletion in the epsilon subunit of the acetylcholine receptor (AChR) in five congenital myasthenic syndrome patients with AChR deficiency. *Ann N Y Acad Sci* **841:** 195–198.

Croxen R, Hatton C, Shelley C et al. (2002) Recessive inheritance and variable penetrance of slow-channel congenital myasthenic syndromes. *Neurology* **59:** 162–168.

Das AS, Agamanolis DP, Cohen BH (2014) Use of next-generation sequencing as a diagnostic tool for congenital myasthenic syndrome. *Pediatr Neurol* **51:** 717–720.

Denning L, Anderson JA, Davis R, Gregg JP, Kuzdenyi J, Maselli RA (2007) High throughput genetic analysis of congenital myasthenic syndromes using resequencing microarrays. *PLoS One* **2:** e918.

Eiden LE (1998) The cholinergic gene locus. *J Neurochem* **70:** 2227–2240.

Engel AG (1988) Congenital myasthenic syndromes. *J Child Neurol* **3:** 233–246.

Engel AG (1994) Congenital myasthenic syndromes. In: Engel AG, Franzini-Armstrong C (Eds), *Myology, Vol I.* New York: McGraw-Hill, pp. 1806–1835.

Engel AG, Lambert EH, Gomez MR (1977) A new myasthenic syndrome with end-plate acetylcholinesterase deficiency, small nerve terminals, and reduced acetylcholine release. *Ann Neurol* **1:** 315–330.

Engel AG, Lambert EH, Mulder DM et al. (1979) Investigations of 3 cases of a newly recognized familial, congenital myasthenic syndrome. *Trans Am Neurol Assoc* **104:** 8–12.

Engel A, Lambert EH, Mulder DM et al. (1981) Recently recognised congenital myasthenic syndromes: clinical features, ultrastructure and cytochemistry. *Ann N Y Acad Sci* **377:** 614–639.

Engel AG, Lambert EH, Mulder DM et al. (1982) A newly recognized congenital myasthenic syndrome attributed to a prolonged open time of the acetylcholine-induced ion channel. *Ann Neurol* **11:** 553–569.

Engel AG, Ohno K, Sine SM (2003) Congenital myasthenic syndromes: progress over the past decade. *Muscle Nerve* **27:** 4–25.

Engel A, Shen X-M, Selcen D, Sine S (2015) Congenital myasthenic syndromes: pathogenesis, diagnosis and treatment. *Lancet Neurol* **14:** 421–434.

Engel AG, Shen XM, Selcen D (2018) The unfolding landscape of the congenital myasthenic syndromes. *Ann N Y Acad Sci* **1413:** 25–34.

Finlayson S, Beeson D, Palace J (2013) Congenital myasthenic syndromes: an update. *Pract Neurol* **13:** 80–91.

Forrest K, Mellerio JE, Robb S, Dopping-Hepenstal PJ, McGrath JA, Liu L et al. (2010) Congenital muscular dystrophy, myasthenic symptoms and epidermolysis bullosa simplex (EBS) associated with mutations in the PLEC1 gene encoding plectin. *Neuromuscul Disord* **20:** 709–711.

Habbout K, Poulin H, Rivier F et al. (2016) A recessive Nav1.4 mutation underlies congenital myasthenic syndrome with periodic paralysis. *Neurology* **86:** 161–169.

Herrmann DN, Horvath R, Sowden JE et al. (2014) Synaptotagmin 2 mutations cause an autosomal dominant form of Lambert–Eaton myasthenic syndrome and non-progressive motor neuropathy. *Am J Hum Genet* **95:** 332–339.

Hoffmann K, Müller JS, Stricker S et al. (2006) Escobar syndrome is a prenatal myasthenia caused by disruption of the acetylcholine receptor fetal γ subunit. *Am J Hum Genet* **79:** 303–312.

Kim N, Stiegler AL, Cameron TO et al. (2008) Lrp4 is a receptor for Agrin and forms a complex with MuSK. *Cell* **135:** 334–342.

Luo S, Cai S, Maxwell S et al. (2017) Novel mutations in the C-terminal region of GMPPB causing limb-girdle muscular dystrophy overlapping with congenital myasthenic syndrome. *Neuromuscul Disord* **27:** 557–564.

Ma C, Su L, Seven AB, Xu Y, Rizo J (2013) Reconstitution of the vital functions of Munc18 and Munc13 in neurotransmitter release. *Science* **339:** 421–425.

Maselli RA, Arredondo J, Cagney O et al. (2010) Mutations in MuSK causing congenital myasthenic syndrome impair MuSK-Dok-7 interaction. *Hum Mol Genet* **19:** 2370–2379.

Maselli RA, Ng JJ, Anderson JA et al. (2009) Mutations in LAMB2 causing a severe form of synaptic congenital myasthenic syndrome. *J Med Genet* **46:** 203–208.

Maselli RA, Arredondo J, Vázquez J et al. (2018) A presynaptic congenital myasthenic syndrome attributed to a homozygous sequence variant in LAMA5. *Ann N Y Acad Sci* **1413:** 119–125.

McMahan UJ, Horton SE, Werle MJ et al. (1992) Agrin isoforms and their role in synaptogenesis. *Curr Opin Cell Biol* **4:** 869–874.

Michalk A, Stricker S, Becker J et al. (2008) Acetylcholine receptor pathway mutations explain various fetal akinesia deformation sequence disorders. *Am J Hum Genet* **82:** 464–476.

Middleton LT (1996) 34th ENMC International Workshop, 10–11 June 1995. Congenital Myasthenic Syndromes. *Neuromuscul Disord* **6:** 133–136.

Mihaylova V, Müller JS, Vilchez JJ et al. (2008) Clinical and molecular genetic findings in COLQ-mutant congenital myasthenic syndromes. *Brain* **131:** 747–759.

Müller JS, Mildner G, Müller-Felber W et al. (2003) Rapsyn N88K is a frequent cause of congenital myasthenic syndromes in European patients. *Neurology* **60:** 1805–1810.

Müller JS, Baumeister SK, Schara U et al. (2006) CHRND mutation causes a congenital myasthenic syndrome by impairing co-clustering of the acetylcholine receptor with rapsyn. *Brain* **129:** 2784–2793.

Nicole S, Chaouch A, Torbergsen T et al. (2014) Agrin mutations lead to a congenital myasthenic syndrome with distal muscle weakness and atrophy. *Brain* **137:** 2429–2443.

O'Connor E, Phan V, Cordts I et al. (2018) MYO9A deficiency in motor neurons is associated with reduced neuromuscular agrin secretion. *Hum Mol Genet* **27:** 1434–1446.

O'Connor E, Töpf A, Müller JS et al. (2016) Identification of mutations in the MYO9A gene in patients with congenital myasthenic syndrome. *Brain* **139:** 2143–2153.

Ohkawara B, Cabrera-Serrano M, Nakata T et al. (2014) LRP4 third β-propeller domain mutations cause novel congenital myasthenia by compromising agrin-mediated MuSK signaling in a position-specific manner. *Hum Mol Genet* **23:** 1856–1868.

Ohno K (2013) Glycosylation defects as an emerging novel cause leading to a limb-girdle type of congenital myasthenic syndromes. *J Neurol Neurosurg Psychiatry* **84:** 1064.

Ohno K, Hutchinson DO, Milone M et al. (1995) Congenital myasthenic syndrome caused by prolonged acetylcholine receptor channel openings due to a mutation in the M2 domain of the epsilon subunit. *Proc Natl Acad Sci USA* **92:** 758–762.

Ohno K, Tsujino A, Brengman JM et al. (2001) Choline acetyltransferase mutations cause myasthenic syndrome associated with episodic apnea in humans. *Proc Natl Acad Sci USA* **98:** 2017–2022.

Okada K, Inoue A, Okada M et al. (2006) The muscle protein Dok-7 is essential for neuromuscular synaptogenesis. *Science* **312:** 1802–1805.

Palace J, Beeson D (2008) The congenital myasthenic syndromes. *J Neuroimmunol* **201–202:** 2–5.

Palace J, Lashley D, Newsom-Davis J et al. (2007) Clinical features of the DOK7 neuromuscular junction synaptopathy. *Brain* **130:** 1507–1515.

Palace J, Lashley D, Bailey S et al. (2012) Clinical features in a series of fast channel congenital myasthenia syndrome. *Neuromuscul Disord* **22:** 112–117.

Pardal-Fernández JM, Carrascosa-Romero MC, Álvarez S, Medina-Monzón MC, Caamaño MB, de Cabo C (2018) A new severe mutation in the SLC5A7 gene related to congenital myasthenic syndrome type 20. *Neuromuscul Disord* **28(10):** 881–884.

Parr JR, Andrew MJ, Finnis M, Beeson D, Vincent A, Jayawant S (2014) How common is childhood myasthenia? The UK incidence and prevalence of autoimmune and congenital myasthenia. *Arch Dis Child* **99:** 539–542.

Pitt MC, Mchugh JC, Deeb J, Smith RA (2017) Assessing neuromuscular junction stability from stimulated EMG in children. *Clin Neurophysiol* **128:** 290–296.

Régal L, Shen X-M, Selcen D et al. (2014) PREPL deficiency with or without cystinuria causes a novel myasthenic syndrome. *Neurology* **82:** 1254–1260.

Robb S, Muntoni F, Simonds A (2010) Respiratory Management of Congenital Myasthenic Syndromes in Childhood: Workshop, 8th December 2009,UCL, Institute of Neurology, London, UK. *Neuromuscul Disord* **20:** 833–838.

Rodríguez Cruz PM, Palace J, Beeson D (2018) The neuromuscular junction and wide heterogeneity of congenital myasthenic syndromes. *Int J Mol Sci* **19(6):** 1677.

Salpietro V, Lin W, Delle Vedove A et al. (2017) Homozygous mutations in VAMP1 cause a presynaptic congenital myasthenic syndrome. *Ann Neurol* **81:** 597–603.

Selcen D, Ohkawara B, Shen X-M, McEvoy K, Ohno K, Engel AG (2015) Impaired synaptic development, maintenance, and neuromuscular transmission in LRP4-related myasthenia. *JAMA Neurol* **72:** 889–896.

Senderek J, Müller JS, Dusl M et al. (2011) Hexosamine biosynthetic pathway mutations cause neuromuscular transmission defect. *Am J Hum Genet* **88:** 162–172.

Schmidt C, Abicht A, Krampfl K et al. (2003) Congenital myasthenic syndrome due to a novel missense mutation in the gene encoding choline acetyltransferase. *Neuromuscul Disord* **13:** 245–251.

Schwartz M, Sternberg D, Whalen S et al. (2018) How chromosomal deletions can unmask recessive mutations? Deletions in 10q11.2 associated with ChAT or SLC18A3 mutations lead to congenital myasthenic syndrome. *Am J Med Genet A* **176:** 151–155.

Shen X-M, Ohno K, Fukudome T et al. (2002) Congenital myasthenic syndrome caused by low-expressor fast-channel AChR delta subunit mutation. *Neurology* **59:** 1881–1888.

Shen X-M, Selcen D, Brengman J, Engel AG (2014) Mutant SNAP25B causes myasthenia, cortical hyperexcitability, ataxia, and intellectual disability. *Neurology* **83:** 2247–2255.

Shen X-M, Scola RH, Lorenzoni PJ et al. (2017) Novel synaptobrevin-1 mutation causes fatal congenital myasthenic syndrome. *Ann Clin Transl Neurol* **4:** 130–138.

Shields MC, Bowers MR, Fulcer MM et al. (2017) Drosophila studies support a role for a presynaptic synaptotagmin mutation in a human congenital myasthenic syndrome. *PLoS One* **12:** e0184817.

Sieb JP, Engel AG (1993) Ephedrine: effects on neuromuscular transmission. *Brain Res* **623:** 167–171.

Sine SM, Ohno K, Bouzat C et al. (1995) Mutation of the acetylcholine receptor alpha subunit causes a slow-channel myasthenic syndrome by enhancing agonist binding affinity. *Neuron* **15**: 229–239.

Slater CR, Fawcett PR, Walls TJ et al. (2006) Pre- and post-synaptic abnormalities associated with impaired neuromuscular transmission in a group of patients with "limb-girdle myasthenia". *Brain* **129**: 2061–2076.

Südhof TC (2013) Neurotransmitter release: the last millisecond in the life of a synaptic vesicle. *Neuron* **80**: 675–690.

Tsujino A, Maertens C, Ohno K et al. (2003) Myasthenic syndrome caused by mutations of the SCN4A sodium channel. *Proc Natl Acad Sci U S A* **100**: 7377–7382.

Whittaker RG, Herrmann DN, Bansagi B et al. (2015) Electrophysiologic features of SYT2 mutations causing a treatable neuromuscular syndrome. *Neurology* **85**: 1964–1971.

Yuste-Checa P, Vega AI, Martín-Higueras C et al. (2017) DPAGT1-CDG: functional analysis of disease-causing pathogenic mutations and role of endoplasmic reticulum stress. *PLoS One* **12**: e0179456.

Zoltowska K, Webster R, Finlayson S et al. (2013) Mutations in GFPT1 that underlie limb-girdle congenital myasthenic syndrome result in reduced cell-surface expression of muscle AChR. *Hum Mol Genet* **22**: 2905–2913.

Drug Treatments in Congenital Myasthenic Syndromes

Sithara Ramdas, Pinki Munot and Stephanie Robb

Congenital myasthenic syndromes (CMS) are rare genetic disorders affecting the integrity of neuromuscular transmission. Currently, mutations in more than 30 genes resulting in CMS have been identified. Symptoms of muscle weakness, fatigue and respiratory crises may be improved and in many cases significantly ameliorated by medications which act at the neuromuscular junction (NMJ) to improve efficiency of neuromuscular transmission. At the outset, it is important to note that drug treatment is usually needed on a life-long basis and is supportive, but not curative. Furthermore, individual genetic subtypes respond to medications acting at the NMJ in differing ways, with drugs that benefit some CMS types proving ineffective or worsening other subtypes (see Table 7.1). It is therefore preferable to have a precise genetic diagnosis before embarking on drug treatment. If this is not possible, then a trial of medication based on the most likely genotype should be given in hospital, with full support facilities available. Currently, there are no licensed drugs for treatment of congenital myasthenia. The drugs used are off-label, the doses and formulations used in CMS may differ from the licensed doses and, hence, these should be initiated and monitored under the supervision of a specialist neurologist with neuromuscular expertise. It is also important to note that certain drugs may take weeks or months before the full response to treatment is apparent.

Although there are no validated paediatric outcome measures to quantify the response, it is important to give adequate thought and consideration to how the response will be measured. Depending on age and motor ability, a combination of baseline physiotherapy measures such as timed rise from the floor, timed 10m run, time to maintain arm forward flexion and up-gaze, repeat sit to stand in 1 minute and 6-minute walk distance (with individual lap times to show fatigue) may be helpful, taken at baseline and repeated at regular follow-up intervals, together with personal/parental reports of changes in functional ability and direct enquiry about possible medication side effects.

A baseline electrocardiogram (ECG) is recommended before commencing 3,4-diaminopyridine (3,4-DAP) (to exclude prolonged QT interval), salbutamol and ephedrine treatment and routine blood pressure monitoring and annual follow-up ECGs are recommended during beta 2 receptor agonist treatment.

DRUGS USED TO TREAT CONGENITAL MYASTHENIC SYNDROMES

The following drugs are used in the treatment of CMS (Table 7.1).

Table 7.1   Drugs for treatment of congenital myasthenic syndromes

Type of congenital myasthenic syndrome	Treatment	Avoid
Acetylcholinesterase deficiency	Salbutamol; ephedrine	Pyridostigmine; 3,4 DAP
Rapsyn	Pyridostigmine; 3,4-DAP; salbutamol	
DOK7	Salbutamol; ephedrine	Pyridostigmine
Acetylcholine receptor deficiency	Pyridostigmine; 3,4-DAP; salbutamol	
Glycosylation (*GFPT1, DAPGT1, ALG2* and *ALG14*)	Pyridostigmine; 3,4 DAP	
ChAT	Pyridostigmine; 3,4-DAP	
COLQ	Ephedrine; salbutamol	
Slow-channel syndrome	Quinidine; fluoxetine	Pyridostigmine
Fast-channel syndrome	Pyridostigmine ± 3,4-DAP	
Agrin/MuSK	May respond to 3,4 DAP	Pyridostigmine
Laminin-β2 deficiency	Ephedrine	Pyridostigmine
LRP4	Salbutamol	
Sodium channele	Pyridostigmine; acetazolamide	
PERPL	Pyridostigmine	
SLC5A7	Pyridostigmine ± 3,4DAP	
Col13A1	3,4DAP ± salbutamol	
Plectin	Pyridostigmine ± 3,4DAP	
SNARE protein complex	3,4DAP; pyridostigmine	

3,4DAP, 3,4diaminopyridine; ChAT, choline acetyl transferase; COLQ, acetylcholinesterase collagenic tail peptide; LRP4, low-density lipoprotein receptor-related protein 4; MuSK, muscle-specific kinase.

Acetylcholinesterase Inhibitors

Acetylcholinesterase inhibitors (AChIs) inhibit the degradation of acetylcholine at the synaptic basal lamina and as a consequence prolong its activity. Pyridostigmine (Mestinon) is most commonly prescribed. The typical dose required is usually 4–7mg/kg/day in four to six divided doses (Engel 2007; Schara and Lochmüller 2008). Higher doses of 7–9mg/kg/day may be required in fast-channel CMS (Lee et al. 2018). Initiation at low dose and gradual increments based on individual response is recommended. Additional doses can be added during periods of increased weakness such as intercurrent illness but it is usual to leave a minimum of 3 hours between each dose. Intramuscular neostigmine (0.5mg/kg) may be used during apnoeic episodes in infants and children (Engel 2007). There is a risk of precipitating cholinergic crisis with AChI, especially at high dosage, although this is usually avoided if the maximum daily dose is kept at or below 7m/kg/day. Side effects may seen at treatment initiation or at high doses. These are mainly cholinergic side effects, including nausea, abdominal cramps, diarrhoea, increased sweating and increased respiratory secretions in infants. Side effects may be controlled by anti-muscarinic agents such as propantheline (Engel et al. 2015; Lee et al. 2018). Careful titration of dose and timing depending on levels of activity during awake periods is often required to achieve maximum benefit. Liquid preparations of AChI are available for younger children, but if children are able to swallow tablets it is more convenient for school/travel to prescribe 60mg tablets, which can be divided with a tablet cutter into half (30mg) or quarter (15mg). These tablets may also be crushed if a liquid preparation is not available. At the time of writing, a long-acting, slow-release AChI preparation is also available, which may be given in the late evening in older children who experience significant weakness in the mornings. Currently, the minimum dose available is 90mg, which precludes usefulness in younger children, who will require smaller doses of AChI.

3,4-Diaminopyridine

3,4-DAP is a potassium channel blocker. It works on the presynaptic nerve terminal by prolonging the motor nerve action potential, and consequently it augments the release of acetylcholine into the synaptic cleft thus enhancing presynaptic transmission (Freeman et al. 1987; Schara and Lochmüller 2008). It works synergistically with AChI (Lee et al. 2018). The recommended dose is up to a maximum of 1mg/kg/day in four divided doses, but lower doses can be efficacious with less side effects (Engel 2007; Schara and Lochmüller 2008; Lee et al. 2018). As recommended above, pretreatment ECG is usually carried out to exclude prolonged QT interval. 3,4-DAP may improve ptosis refractory to pyridostigmine. A common side effect, especially at higher doses is perioral and peripheral paraesthesiae. Hyperactivity and insomnia can be an additional feature in young children. Seizures have been reported as a rare but serious side effects of 3,4-DAP when used in the treatment of Lambert–Eaton myasthenic syndrome, although the risk is thought to be dose dependent (Lindquist and Stangel 2011). As a result, caution is advised in using 3,4-DAP if there is any history of seizures and, if necessary, a baseline electroencephalography carried out before starting 3,4-DAP.

Beta-2 Receptor Agonists

These include ephedrine and salbutamol (Albuterol). The exact mechanism of action of these at the NMJ is not fully understood, but it is thought they stabilise the structure of the NMJ and reduce the dispersion of AChR (Beeson 2016). They stabilise motor endplate structures through activation of second messenger signalling (Burke et al. 2013). As the effect on the structure of the NMJ is gradual, the response to treatment is not immediate and is seen over several months and some cases may continue to improve even 12 months after initiating treatment (Cruz et al. 2015). Oral salbutamol (Albuterol) is generally well tolerated. Side effects include muscle cramps (especially with DOK7 CMS) hypertension, tachycardia and hypokalemia (especially during intercurrent illness), particularly at higher doses. Investigations including ECG, blood pressure and plasma potassium level are recommended prior to initiation and at regular follow-up intervals and also during periods of decompensation during intercurrent illness. The prescribed dose of salbutamol (Albuterol) ranges from 0.1mg/kg/day three times daily (up to a maximum of 2mg/dose) for children aged less than 6 years, 2mg/dose 2–3 times daily for children between ages 6–12 years, and 4–8mg/dose 1–3 times daily more than 12 years and in adults (Leiwluck et al. 2011). Ephedrine may be used as an alternative to salbutamol, although is currently unavailable in some countries. The initial oral dose of ephedrine of 1mg/kg/day for children, divided into three doses per day, and is gradually increased to a maximum of 3mg/kg/day (Schara and Lochmüller 2008). The adult oral dose is 25–50mg, administered 2–3 times daily (Bestue-Cardiel et al. 2005; Engel 2007; Schara and Lochmüller 2008). Ephedrine, even in low dosage, may cause irritability in infants and high doses should be prescribed with caution because of possible adverse effects, such as hypertension, anxiety, insomnia, and palpitations (Schara and Lochmüller 2008).

Fluoxetine and Quinidine

Fluoxetine and quinidine reduce the duration of opening of the AChR ion channel (Sieb et al. 1996; Harper and Engel 1998; Harper et al. 2003; Beeson et al. 2005; Engel 2007; Schara and Lochmüller 2008). As a result they prevent the depolarisation block and desensitisation of AChR at physiologic rates of stimulation and mitigate the cationic overloading of the postsynaptic region and its sequelae. There is no

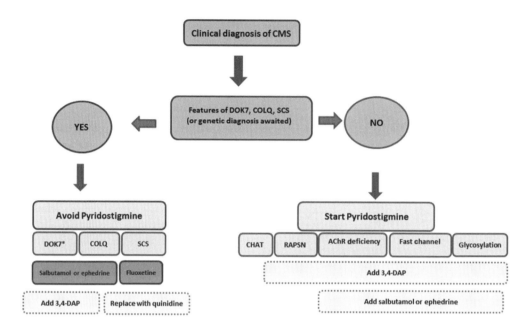

Figure 7.1   Treatment algorithm for the common CMS subtypes. First-line treatment: boxes with continuous lines. Second-/third-line treatments: boxes with dotted lines. DOK7, downstream of tyrosine kinase 7; COLQ, acetylcholinesterase collagenic tail peptide; SCS, slow channel congenital myasthenic sydrome; CHAT, choline acetyltransferase; RAPSN, receptor associated protein of the synapse; AChR, acetylcholine receptor; 3,4-DAP, 3,4-diaminopyridine. Reproduced from Lee (2018) with permission from Wiley.

clear evidence of superiority of either drug in slow-channel CMS. Quinidine can cause cardiac conduction defects. Fluoxetine can prolong the QT interval at high doses and there is risk of suicidal ideation in children and adolescents and should be used only under psychiatric supervision (Harper and Engel 1998; Harper et al. 2003; Lee et al. 2018). Cholinesterase inhibitors should be avoided in slow-channel CMS because they may exacerbate endplate myopathy and cause clinical deterioration (Sieb et al. 1996; Beeson et al. 2004; Lorenzoni et al. 2006).

As previously mentioned, it is important to recognise that drugs beneficial in one type of CMS can be ineffective or harmful in another type. For example, patients AChR deficiency or fast-channel mutations in AChR subunits improve with cholinergic agonists, whereas patients with slow-channel mutations, *COLQ* and *DOK7* mutations can deteriorate. Therefore genetic diagnosis and molecular pathology should inform the choice of therapy. When genetic diagnosis is not available, therapeutic trials should be tailored to the most likely genetic defect based on the clinical phenotype. The following table and flowchart provide a suggested therapeutic regime in the genetic subtypes of CMS. It is also important to recognise that pyridostigmine and 3,4-DAP exert an immediate effect whereas the effect of adrenergic agonists and quinidine/fluoxetine is slow, over weeks or months (Fig. 7.1).

OTHER MANAGEMENT

In addition to drug treatment, children with CMS have complex medical needs which require the input of a multi-disciplinary team. Some aspects of these will be discussed in detail in other chapters in the book including respiratory management and physiotherapy. Other important interventions are outlined in the following sections.

Speech and Language Therapy

Children with significant bulbar difficulties require feeding via nasogastric tube or percutaneous gastrostomy. In addition, even those with normal or mildly abnormal bulbar function may require texture modifications or artificial feeding during intercurrent illnesses. Speech difficulties especially articulation difficulties are not uncommon and require the expertise of a speech and language therapist.

Education

Children with CMS have normal cognition but due to their physical difficulties will struggle to access the full curriculum. It is important that children are well supported at school so they are not at disadvantage due to their CMS. Simple measure like appropriate seating position in the classroom or access to a laptop can be prevent fatigue. The variable nature of the condition in a child during a single day, week or periods of intercurrent illness can be challenging for schools to understand and manage. Hence, close liaison with school by the local therapist or a neuromuscular nurse specialist is recommended. Periods of rest especially during physical education will reduce falls and injuries resulting from muscle fatigue. Classes on lower levels may help with ease of access to a full curriculum and also enhance safety. Help may be needed with feeding and toileting in the school. Use of a laptop and extra time for timed tests during exams may need to be requested.

Social Care

As with all children with complex medical needs, social care involvement is essential for several reasons including appropriate housing, financial and social support for parents and siblings. House adaptations and modifications may be needed. Transport especially to and from school will need to be arranged. Carers may need flexible job opportunities to be able to look after their children and carers allowance as well as respite care for the family needs to be considered.

Nutrition and Feeding

This may pose a significant challenge with inadequate nutrition and safety of swallowing being compromised. Nasogastric tube feeding and sometimes percutaneous gastrostomy (PEG) feeds may be needed to ensure adequate and safe feeding.

Therapy

Children with CMS will need ongoing physiotherapy to prevent contractures. Exercise to build up some degree of fitness is to be encouraged and immobility discouraged. Some exercise has been shown to slow development of weakness and muscle atrophy and can sometimes improve muscle strength as well. Development of scoliosis needs monitoring. Adequate seating, bracing, shoes and appliances may be required to help with everyday function. Wheelchairs and supports in the chair will need to be reviewed by wheelchair services accessed through the occupational therapy services who can also assist with home adaptations.

Respiratory Function

This needs monitoring as well as looking for signs of respiratory failure. Flu vaccination in the winter months should be offered. Some children may need constant suctioning or use of a non-invasive ventilator and cough assist machines.

REFERENCES

Beeson D (2016) Congenital myasthenic syndromes: recent advances. *Curr Opin Neurol* **29**: 565–571.

Beeson D, Hantaï D, Lochmüller H, Engel AG (2005) 126th International Workshop: Congenital Myasthenic Syndromes, 24–26 September 2004, Naarden, the Netherlands. *Neuromuscul Disord* **15**: 498–512.

Bestue-Cardiel M, Cabezon-Alvarez AS, Capablo-Liesa JL et al. (2005) Congenital endplate acetylcholinesterase deficiency responsive to ephedrine. *Neurology* **65**: 144–146.

Burke G, Hiscock A, Klein A et al. (2013) Salbutamol benefits children with congenital myasthenic syndrome due to DOK7 mutations. *Neuromuscul Disord* **23**: 170–175.

Engel AG (2007) The therapy of congenital myasthenic syndromes. *Neurotherapeutics* **4**: 252–257.

Engel AG, Shen XM, Selcen D, Sine SM (2015) Congenital myasthenic syndromes: pathogenesis, diagnosis, and treatment. *Lancet Neurol* **14**: 420–434.

Freeman GB, Mykytyn V, Gibson GE (1987) Differential alteration of dopamine, acetylcholine, and glutamate release during anoxia and/or 3,4-diaminopyridine treatment. *Neurochem Res* **12**: 1019–1027.

Harper CM, Engel AG (1998) Quinidine sulphate therapy for the slow-channel congenital myasthenic syndrome. *Ann Neurol* **43**: 480–484.

Harper CM, Fukodome T, Engel AG (2003) Treatment of slow-channel congenital myasthenic syndrome with fluoxetine. *Neurology* **60**: 1710–1713.

Lee M, Beeson D, Palace J (2018) Therapeutic strategies for congenital myasthenic syndromes. *Ann N Y Acad Sci* **1412**: 129–136.

Liewluck T, Selcen D, Engel AG (2011) Beneficial effects of albuterol in congenital endplate acetylcholinesterase deficiency and Dok-7 myasthenia. *Muscle Nerve* **44**: 789–794.

Lindquist S, Stangel M (2011) Update on treatment options for Lambert–Eaton myasthenic syndrome: focus on use of amifampridine. *Neuropsychiatr Dis Treat* **7**: 341–349.

Lorenzoni PJ, Kay CS, Arruda WO, Scola RH, Werneck LC (2006) [Neurophysiological study in slow-channel congenital myasthenic syndrome: case report]. *Arq Neuropsiquiatr* **64(2A)**: 318–321.

Palace J, Lashley D, Bailey S et al. (2012) Clinical features in a series of fast channel congenital myasthenia syndrome. *Neuromuscul Disord* **22**: 112–117.

Rodríguez Cruz PM, Palace J, Ramjattan H, Jayawant S, Robb SA, Beeson D (2015) Salbutamol and ephedrine in the treatment of severe AChR deficiency syndromes. *Neurology* **85**: 1043–1047.

Schara U, Lochmüller H (2008) Therapeutic strategies in congenital myasthenic syndromes. *Neurotherapeutics* **5**: 542–547.

Sieb JP, Milone M, Engel AG (1996) Effects of the quinoline derivatives quinine, quinidine, and chloroquine on neuromuscular transmission. *Brain Res* **712**: 179–189.

Neuromuscular Disorders with Transmission Defects

Vamshi K Rao and Nancy L Kuntz

INTRODUCTION

Neuromuscular junction (NMJ) development starts with polyneuronal innervation – one Schwann cell covering several axons over a single muscle endplate. Beginning at 17–20 weeks of gestation, this simple structure starts to become complex with the appearance of secondary clefts. The junctional folds then deepen and acquire densely packed acetylcholine receptors (AChRs) in the postsynaptic membrane (Fidziańska 1980). It is not entirely known whether there is an inherent defect in the embryonic development of this NMJ in neuromuscular disorders or whether decreased movement leads to remodelling and degeneration.

Muscle inactivity has been demonstrated in several animal studies to cause defects in NMJ maturation and NMJ degeneration (Benoit and Changeux 1975; Thompson et al. 1979; Brenner et al. 1987; Fahim 1989). Inactivity was also shown to be the reason for an NMJ defect in a baby with X-linked centronuclear myopathy (XL-CNM) who had electromyography (EMG) features of muscle denervation (Elder et al. 1983). Cholinesterase staining was used in this instance to demonstrate small muscle end plates and normal nerve terminals. An elaborate study of the ultrastructure of the NMJ in this extremely inactive baby showed the presence of neural cell adhesion molecule (N-CAM) positive myotubes. The presence of such myotubes suggested that the myofibres were arrested in maturation and anomalous nerve-muscle contacts led to endplate remodelling manifested by degeneration and regeneration (Fidziańska and Goebel 1994). Alternatively, one could propose that genes implicated in neuromuscular disorders are also required for maintenance and function of an otherwise normally developed junctional structure.

NEUROMUSCULAR TRANSMISSION ABNORMALITIES IN MOTOR NEURON DISORDERS

Neuromuscular transmission defects, as evidenced by decrement on repetitive nerve stimulation, have been demonstrated in individuals with motor neuron disease, such as progressive muscular atrophy and amyotrophic lateral sclerosis (ALS) in multiple studies (Killian et al. 1994; Iwanami et al. 2011; Kim et al. 2011). Animal models of ALS have uncovered the loss of the synapse and decreased axonal sprouting, lending credence to the defect in transmission across the NMJ (Frey et al. 2000; Rocha et al. 2013; Shahidullah et al. 2013). Defects are also seen with respect to quantal release, leading to failure of synaptic transmission before motor neuronal degeneration and/or overt motor symptoms (Kariya et al. 2008;

Kong et al. 2009; Armstrong and Drapeau 2013; Rocha et al. 2013). In the TDP-43 ALS mouse model, NMJ pathology seemed to precede development of motor deficits associated with the disease (Chand et al. 2018).

Spinal Muscular Atrophy

Spinal muscular atrophy (SMA) is an autosomal recessive disorder of childhood. In the most common form, it is due to a homozygous deletion of survival motor neuron 1 (*SMN*) gene located on chromosome 5. The number of copies of the alternatively spliced homologue, *SMN2*, influences disease phenotype. Natural history studies reveal three common childhood phenotypes, type 1 where babies do not attain the ability to sit; type 2, where children sit but do not walk; and type 3 children walk independently but gait is abnormal, and ambulation can be progressively lost over time (Lunn and Wang 2008; Kolb and Kissel 2011).

SMN has been found to have a role in not only motor neuron in development but also in NMJ maturation (Bowerman et al. 2012). SMN protein has an important role in neurite outgrowth and neuromuscular maturation (Fan and Simard 2002). SMN deficiency leading to defects in neuromuscular maturation and development has been studied extensively as a process contributing to the pathogenesis of SMA.

Animal models with SMN deficiency demonstrate both pre- and postsynaptic junction pathology (Kariya et al. 2008; Murray et al. 2008). There is a decreased number of synaptic vesicles at the nerve terminal with impaired release and accumulation of abnormal neurofilaments (Kong et al. 2009).

Ling et al. (2012), using SMNΔ7 mice, showed severe denervation (<50% fully innervated endplates) in many axial muscles and appendicular muscles at end stage of disease. These muscles are initially innervated but then undergo denervation resulting in loss of NMJ maintenance. Antisense oligonucleotides (ASO) have been used in mouse models of SMA to ameliorate the genetic defect and increase SMN protein. Treatment of these mice with ASO therapy significantly reversed the NMJ denervation in those muscles and increased survival (Lin et al. 2016).

In a study by Arnold et al. (2004), using cells of patients with SMA type 1, myoblasts were shown to fuse, albeit abnormally, to form immature myotubes. These myotubes had few nuclei and abnormal nicotinic acetyl choline receptor (nAChR) aggregation. There was shown to be diminished expression of nAChR protein. The study concluded that the earliest defect in NMJ development is due to the postsynaptic muscle component and that the NMJs may be installed early in development but lack the capacity to function due to a postsynaptic defect thereby contributing to disease pathogenesis.

NMJ function was investigated by Wadman et al. (2012) in SMA patients by repetitive nerve stimulation (RNS); 35 patients were compared to 20 healthy controls and five controls with motor neuron disease. Significant decrement (>10%) was seen in 49% of individuals with type 2 and 3 SMA without any abnormal increment (>60%) on RNS. Controls, both healthy and with motor neuron disease, did not show any decrement. The decrement without an incremental response to RNS supported the hypothesis of a postsynaptic defect in SMA. The study did not find a correlation between decreased compound muscle action potential (CMAP) amplitudes at baseline and decrement. The decrement was more frequent in individuals with early-onset disease suggesting that SMN protein concentration may be below a critical threshold level required for normal NMJ development and maintenance. Four patients took pyridostigmine at doses of 4mg/kg for several days and, of those, two reported increased stamina.

RNS was also used as a technique to demonstrate neuromuscular transmission (NMT) defects in SMA patients by Preterre et al. (2015). The group selected eight SMA patients (two type 2 and five type 3) and compared them to eight control volunteers. All the SMA patients chosen had complained that their motor disability increased as the day progressed. RNS (3Hz) was performed by stimulating the hypoglossal, radial and accessory nerve and recording over the genioglossus, anconeus and trapezius muscles respectively. Significant decrement (>10%) was observed in at least one muscle-nerve territory in 75% patients versus none in healthy controls (p<0.003). The accessory nerve stimulation recording over the trapezius was the more sensitive test.

Spinal and Bulbar Muscular Atrophy

Spinal and bulbar muscular atrophy (SBMA) also known as Kennedy disease is a rare (1 in 150 000 males), slowly progressive neuromuscular condition with onset in males between ages of 20–50 years. Bulbar weakness with dysphagia in addition to other features, such as muscle cramps and gynecomastia, is seen. Most of these symptoms are postulated to be due to a loss of alpha motor neurons in the spinal and bulbar regions. One of the proposed mechanisms of SBMA involves the muscle as the trigger of dysfunction, which in a retrograde fashion then disturbs the NMJ and ultimately results in motor neuron death (Ferri et al. 2003; Brady and Morfini 2010). The NMJ has been shown to be fragmented (Kemp et al. 2011) and demonstrate abnormal synaptic vesicle staining (Katsuno et al. 2006) in animal models.

Xu et al. (2016) utilising three adult SBMA mouse models studied synaptic function by recording the miniature and evoked endplate potentials (miniature endplate potential [MEPP] and EPP respectively) intracellularly from the muscle fibres. Neurophysiologic recordings by Xu et al. demonstrate that there is decrease in the overall quantal content presynaptically with the signals having a prolonged decay time postsynaptically. Furthermore, quantitative PCR revealed an upregulation of the neonatal form of AChR.

NEUROMUSCULAR TRANSMISSION ABNORMALITIES IN MUSCULAR DYSTROPHIES

Myotonic Dystrophy Type 1

Myotonic dystrophy (DM1) is an autosomal dominant disorder that results from a trinucleotide, CTG, repeat in the *DMPK* gene on chromosome 19q.13.3. In the congenital form repeats of over 1000 are encountered. Disease manifestations include myotonia, muscle weakness with systemic and bulbar symptoms along with involvement of the brain, heart, eye, respiratory, endocrine, gastro-intestinal and integumentary systems (Bird 1993).

Nerve excitability studies in DM1 with looking at maximal contraction demonstrated increased excitability in patients with myotonic dystrophy as compared to controls. These findings hypothesised that threshold recovery time is lengthened after maximal contraction and likely contributed to fatigue in DM1 (Krishnan and Kiernan 2006).

Abnormal splicing causing decreased conductance of chloride and changes in the insulin receptor signalling may affect the stability and function of the NMJ in DM1 (Wheeler et al. 2007). NMJ abnormalities on histopathology of patient specimens, both with light and electron microscopy techniques, have been shown (MacDermot 1961). Furthermore, NMJ involvement in respiratory and diaphragmatic dysfunction was also reported in a transgenic mice model of DM1 (Panaite et al. 2008).

Repetitive motor conduction study done on three individuals (23–56 years) with myotonic dystrophy at 5 and 10Hz stimulation showed 20–52% decrement (Aminoff et al. 1977). To further test NMJ neurophysiological abnormalities in patients with DM1, Bombelli et al. (2016) performed RNS and SFEMG. Standard nerve conduction studies (NCS) were normal in all patients. Approximately 28% (4/14) of DM1 individuals showed abnormal decrement ranging from 12–20% on 3Hz RNS whereas 71% (10/14) had abnormal jitter and blocking. All controls had normal RNS and single fibre EMG (SFEMG) values (Bombelli et al. 2016).

Duchenne Muscular Dystrophy

Duchenne muscular dystrophy (DMD) is a disorder that has progressive course of skeletal muscle weakness along with cardiac muscle involvement that is fatal mostly before the third decade of life (Birnkrant et al. 2018). The disorder is due to absence of dystrophin protein. Dystrophin function is to stabilise the muscle fibre by connecting the extracellular and transmembrane protein cluster to the intracellular and actin complex. The complex, postsynaptically, is enriched at the NMJ by the presence of utrophin, a homologue of dystrophin that is otherwise absent extrasynaptically (Blake et al. 2002). Since utrophin null mice are phenotypically normal and have normal AChR histology, a model deficient in both dystrophin and utrophin (mdx/utrn$^{-/-}$) was proposed, as these mice die in 4–14 weeks, have severe weakness and demonstrated punctate AChR clusters (Deconinck et al. 1997; Grady et al. 1997).

A comprehensive study involving mice with both dystrophin and utrophin deficiency genotypes was undertaken (van der Pijl et al. 2016). Inverted mesh and grip strength testing showed reduced muscle strength and increased fatigability in the dystrophic mice. The force of pull with successive trials of grip strength waned in the dystrophic mouse models. Electrodecrement was noted at 40Hz stimulation in mdx/utrn$^{+/-}$ and mdx/utrn$^{-/-}$ mice compared with wild type, and the decrement was most pronounced in mdx/utrn$^{-/-}$ mice. EPP decrement was more pronounced in the dystrophic mice; in addition, they had lowered postsynaptic ACh sensitivity, both these effects negatively impacting the safety factor of neuromuscular transmission. AChR fragmentation was noted at the NMJs of all the DMD mouse models when compared to wild type but did not reach statistical significance. The study concludes that NMJs of all three DMD mouse models used, showed functional pathologies resulting in decreased safety factor of neuromuscular transmission. The reduced safety factor might lead to neuromuscular transmission failure especially during increased activity. This may be more relevant in DMD patients as the safety factor is even lower in humans (Wood and Slater 2001) and the muscle damage is more severe compared to mice, leading to more intense strain on the remaining fibres, to sustain function (van der Pijl et al. 2016). All these findings may bring to the foreground the possible use of drugs enhancing neuromuscular transmission across the NMJ.

NEUROMUSCULAR TRANSMISSION ABNORMALITIES IN MYOPATHIES

Mitochondrial Myopathies

Mitochondrial gene mutations can lead to a spectrum of disorders with variable neurological presentations including neuromuscular phenotypes such as myopathy and neuropathy (McFarland et al. 2010). There has however been paucity in the literature about defects in neuromuscular transmission with these gene defects.

Recently, a mitochondrial citrate carrier *SLC25A1* was reported to cause agenesis of corpus callosum and optic nerve hypoplasia by one group (Edvardson et al. 2013). This child was noted to have poor suck, and recurrent apnoeas. Later, cognitive delays, seizures and decreased spontaneous movements were seen. A SFEMG demonstrated significantly increased jitter and blocking but symptoms did not fluctuate. In addition, there was no improvement with pyridostigmine, 3,4-DAP or ephedrine.

Chaouch and co-workers found an *SLC25A1* variant in a case of siblings who were diagnosed as congenital myasthenia and were responsive to medication (Chaouch et al. 2014). The siblings were born to consanguineous parents from the north of England. The index patient was a 33-year-old male who had intermittent leg weakness in early childhood that improved with rest. He has mild ptosis in both eyes and dysarthria. There was presence of fatigable weakness. The 19-year-old sister had more delayed cognitive and motor milestones compared to the brother, and fell frequently in infancy. She had diplopia and clear fatigable weakness. RNS performed in the brother in his 20s did not show decrement but SFEMG was abnormal with increased jitter and blocking. The brother did not benefit from use of pyridostigmine, but 3,4-DAP helped.

The authors then proceeded to study a defect in neuromuscular transmission in zebrafish. They used antisense morpholino oligonucleotides to knock down the two zebrafish *SLC25A1* orthologs. Knockdown in zebrafish embryos manifested itself by alteration in tail morphology and swimming behaviours. The presentation is reminiscent of a knock down of NMJ proteins. Furthermore, histological analysis of the affected embryos was of a presynaptic defect with short motor terminals and incomplete synapse formation.

CONGENITAL MYOPATHIES

Congenital myopathies are a clinically and genetically heterogeneous group of disorders characterised by weakness, hypotonia with onset usually at birth and a slowly progressive course (North 2011). Historically, congenital myopathies were defined by histopathological features on muscle biopsy. Over the last two decades a number of genetic mutations have been shown to be causative (Cassandrini et al. 2017; Kress et al. 2017). In the last decade, a variety of animal models and case reports have been published demonstrating neuromuscular transmission defects in congenital myopathies (Rodríguez Cruz et al. 2014).

Nemaline Myopathies

Nemaline myopathies are a group of clinically heterogeneous disorders that are characterised pathologically by the presence of typical rod-like structures in the muscle fibre called nemaline bodies (Wallgren-Pettersson et al. 2011). Clinical presentation can range from mild-to-severe muscle weakness. To date, nine different mutations have been identified with nemaline rod myopathy: *ACTA1, NEB, TPM2, TPM3, TNNT1, CFL2, KBTBD13, KLHL40, KLHL41.*

KLHL40

Kelch-like family member mutations (*KLHL40* and *KLH41*) are associated with a severe clinical phenotype of nemaline myopathy with fetal akinesia, respiratory difficulties, swallowing issues, multiple joint contractures, fractures and dysmorphic features at birth (Ravenscroft et al. 2013; Kawase et al. 2015). A case report of a child with a the *KLHL40* mutation illustrates the severity of presentation followed by remarkable improvement with use of acetylcholinesterase inhibitors (ACEI) and later, the added beneficial effect of ephedrine. This child was a female born to a consanguineous couple with polyhydramnios and fetal bradykinesia who demonstrated severe muscle weakness, with no spontaneous antigravity movements at birth, requiring intubation. She needed invasive respiratory support and nasogastric tube feedings even at 1 year of age when ptosis was noted. This led to a therapeutic trial of pyridostigmine at 20mg/kg/day (Natera-de Benito et al. 2016). Within 3 days of treatment, she showed remarkable improvement with spontaneous movements and increase in facial expression. With continued treatment, she was sitting unassisted after 2 months, walking with support after 6 months and after 18 months (2.5yrs of age) walking independently. An addition of ephedrine (30mg daily) to the ACEI regimen led to improvement in walking distance and decreased rise from floor time. Histopathological and genetic work-up led to a diagnosis of *KLHL40* nemaline myopathy. At the last report the child was 9 years of age with normal cognitive and academic development, on pyridostigmine 20mg/kg/day and ephedrine 50mg daily. There had been no progression of weakness, ambulation was preserved but a persistence of bulbar weakness and speech/swallowing dysfunction necessitated continuance of nasogastric tube feeding.

Centronuclear Myopathies

Centronuclear myopathies (CNM) are a group of genetically and clinically diverse disorders that share a common histopathology comprising central nuclei in the muscle fibres without necrosis or regeneration.

Mutations in multiple genes reveal central nuclei on biopsy with *MTM1*, *DNM2*, *BIN1*, *RYR1*, *DM1* mutations comprising 70% of published cases (Romero 2010). There are several reports of myasthenic features with fatigable weakness, electrophysiological abnormalities and improvement with use of ACEIs in children with centronuclear myopathy.

X-linked Myotubular Myopathy

A male child with features of myotubular myopathy (MTM) and confirmed mutation in the exon 9 of the *MTM1* gene has been reported. His motor abilities declined after 13 years of age to the point where he was extremely fatigued and able to walk only with support. SFEMG revealed mildly increased jitter in the orbicularis oculi. A trial of pyridostigmine 30mg once daily increased his exercise tolerance and he was walking longer, albeit with assistance. Pyridostigmine was discontinued due to abdominal pain and diarrhoea resulting in decline in motor function with inability to weight bear. Gradual re-establishment of pyridostigmine (up to 45mg daily) increased his strength again with standing ability for transfers and increase in swimming distance (Robb et al. 2011).

Dynamin 2 Myopathy

Five cases have been reported with mutations in the dynamin 2 (*DNM2*) gene showing clinical features of neuromuscular transmission defect and improvement with ACEI (Gibbs et al. 2013).

Centronuclear Myopathies with Unidentified Genes

Robb et al. (2011) describe three individuals with NMT defects whose muscle biopsy was consistent with centronuclear myopathy (CNM).

Bridging Integrator 1/Amphiphysin 2

A male child born to a Moroccan family demonstrated ptosis, dysarthria, delayed motor milestones (walked at 3.5 yrs. of age) and difficulty running. He also had mild cognitive delay. Progressive weakness ensued from 3.5 years of age with proximal and distal weakness, scapular winging, frequent falls and fatigability. AChR and muscle-specific kinase (MuSK) antibody testing was negative; 3Hz RNS showed decrement of 14–30%. Muscle biopsy showed features of CNM and genetic testing revealed a missense mutation in bridging integrator 1 gene (*BIN1*) (Claeys et al. 2010).

Congenital Fibre Type Disproportion

Congenital fibre type disproportion (CFTD) is a congenital myopathy with clinical and genetically heterogeneous presentation characterised by type 1 fibre hypotrophy and relative type 2 hypertrophy (Sewry 2008). Mutations in six genes (*ACTA1*, *TPM3*, *TPM2*, *RYR1*, *SEPN1*, *MYH7*) have been implicated to date. CFTD usually presents with hypotonia and mild-to-severe muscle weakness at birth or within the first year of life. The majority of these children eventually develop the ability to walk. Muscle weakness is static in more than 90% of individuals. Respiratory failure, ophthalmoplegia, ptosis, and facial and/or bulbar weakness usually predict poor prognosis (Clarke and North 2003).

Tropomyosin 3

Two cases have been reported to have mutations in the tropomyosin 3 (*TPM3*) gene with clinicopathological features of CFTD and defects in NMT (Munot et al. 2010). In the first child, muscle biopsy at 11 years of age revealed type 1 fibre hypotrophy with no nemaline rods. Stimulated SFEMG showed increased jitter. A trial of salbutamol at age 15 produced no benefit but a trial of pyridostigmine and 3,4-DAP

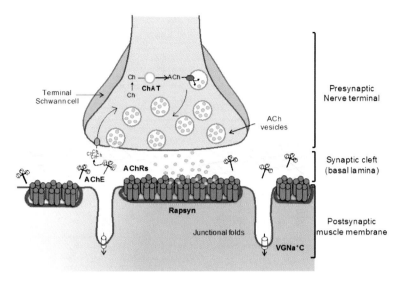

Figure 1.1 Schematic representation of the neuromuscular junction. The NMJ is divided into three different compartments. The presynaptic nerve terminal is responsible for the synthesis (ChAT) and recycling of acetylcholine and the exocytosis of synaptic vesicles. The synaptic cleft contains a specialised form of extracellular matrix called basal lamina that is essential for the structural integrity of the NMJ. This the location of the enzyme AChE, which breaks down ACh into Ch. At the postsynaptic muscle compartment, the AChRs are densely clustered at the top of the junctional folds forming a network with the intracellular anchoring protein rapsyn that stabilises AChRs (Zuber and Unwin 2013). VGNa+C located at the bottom of the junctional folds are essential in the generation and propagation of action potentials. ACh, acetylcholine; AChE, acetylcholinesterase; AChR, acetylcholine receptor; Ch, choline; ChAT, choline acetyltransferase; NMJ, neuromuscular junction; VGNa+C, voltage-gated sodium channel.

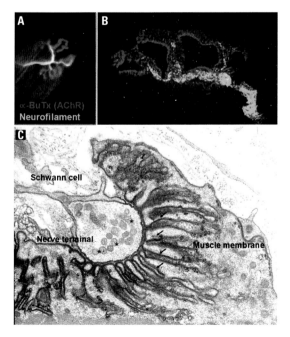

Figure 1.2 Fluorescence and electron microscopy images of the neuromuscular junction. A Fluorescence microscopy image of the NMJ showing the nerve terminal (green) innervating the muscle endplate (red) stained with fluorescently conjugated α-bungarotoxin that binds to the AChRs. **B** Super-resolution confocal microscopy image of the NMJ showing the postsynaptic muscle membrane and the junctional folds at the top of which AChRs are concentrated (image provided by Dr J. Cheung). **C** Electron microscopy image of the NMJ. The presynaptic nerve terminal is filled with synaptic vesicles containing acetylcholine (*). The postsynaptic muscle membrane exhibits a high degree of folding which extends into the muscle sarcoplasm (arrows) in order to increase the total endplate surface. The NMJ is covered by terminal Schwann cells. AChR, acetylcholine receptor; NMJ, neuromuscular junction. Adapted from Slater (2017) with permission.

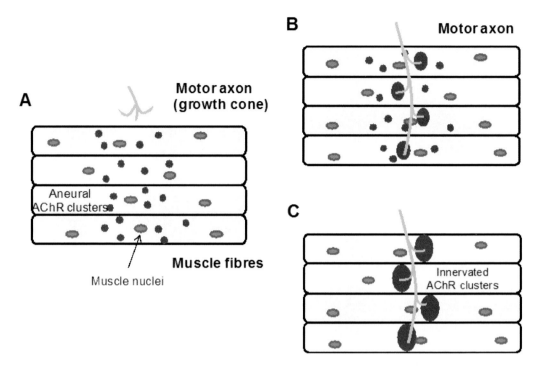

Figure 1.3 Schematic representation of the neuromuscular junction development. A Aneural AChR clusters are prepatterned in the midbelly of the muscle fibres prior to the arrival of the nerve terminal. **B** Upon innervation of the prepatterned clusters in the synaptic region, they become enlarged while aneural clusters located in the extrasynaptic region disappear. **C** As a result, AChR clusters are concentrated at a high density in the area underneath the nerve terminal maximising the efficiency of neuromuscular transmission. AChR, acetylcholine receptor. Adapted from Lin et al. (2001) with permission from Springer Nature.

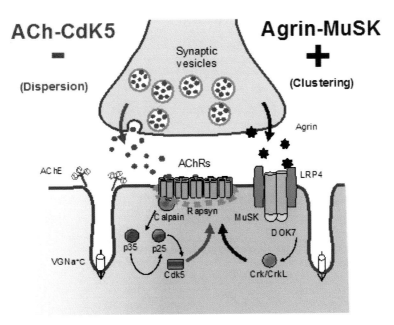

Figure 1.4   Schematic representation the neuromuscular junction and the acetylcholine receptor clustering and dispersal pathways. Upon the release of agrin by the nerve terminal, agrin binds to LRP4 resulting in MuSK dimerisation and activation (Kim et al. 2008). This leads to the recruitment of DOK7 (Okada et al. 2006), a muscle-specific cytoplasmic adaptor of MuSK that further stimulates MuSK activation propagating the signal downstream which results in the clustering of the AChRs by the cytoplasmic anchoring protein rapsyn. By contrast, ACh is believed to disperse AChR clusters through a cyclin-dependent kinase (CdK5) mechanism linked to the interaction of rapsyn and the calcium-dependent protease calpain (Chen et al. 2007). Calpain activity promotes the cleavage of p35 to p25 (Patrick et al. 1999), an activator of CdK5. Rapsyn is believed to stabilise AChR clusters by suppressing calpain activity. ACh, acetylcholine; AChR, acetylcholine receptor; LRP4, low-density lipoprotein receptor 4; MuSK, muscle-specific kinase; VGNa+C, voltage-gated Na+ channel. Adapted from Rodriguez Cruz et al. (2018) with permission.

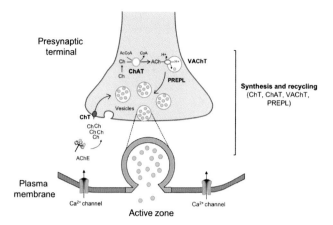

Figure 1.5 Schematic representation of the nerve terminal and the main molecules involved in the synthesis and recycling of acetylcholine. In the synaptic cleft, AChE breaks down acetylcholine (ACh) into acetate and Ch, which is uptaken by the ChT to the presynaptic terminal. The enzyme ChAT catalyses the synthesis of ACh from AcCoA and choline, and the vesicular acetylcholine transporter VAChT loads ACh into synaptic vesicles. *PREPL* encodes a protein thought to be involved in the trafficking of VAChT. AcCoA, acetyl coenzyme A; ACh, acetylcholine; AChE, acetylcholinesterase; AChR, acetylcholine receptor; Ch, choline; ChAT, choline acetyltransferase; ChT, sodium-dependent high-affinity choline transporter 1; NMJ, neuromuscular junction; VAChT, vesicular acetylcholine transporter; VGNa+C, voltage-gated sodium channel.

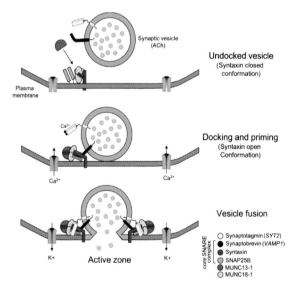

Figure 1.6 Schematic representation of synaptic vesicles at the active zones of presynaptic terminals. The influx of Ca^{2+} following an action potential causes synaptic vesicles to fuse to the plasma membrane through SNARE proteins (synaptobrevin, syntaxin and SNAP25B) releasing the neurotransmitter acetylcholine to the synaptic cleft (Chen and Scheller 2001). The calcium current persists until the membrane potential is returned to normal by outward fluxes of potassium. Munc18-1 is a chaperone that binds to a self-inhibited "closed" conformation of syntaxin-1B and to SNARE complexes (Lai et al. 2017). Munc13-1, is believed to be involved in synaptic vesicle priming prior to vesicle fusion by catalysing the transition of syntaxin 1B from a closed configuration with Munc18-1 into an open state ready to form SNARE complexes and fuse rapidly. The core SNARE complex, a 4-α helix structure formed by the synaptic vesicle-associated synaptobrevin (v-SNARE) and the presynaptic SNAP25B and syntaxin 1B (t-SNARES) proteins, brings the vesicle and plasma membranes together. Finally, calcium-bound Synaptotagmin (a vesicle Ca^{2+} sensor) binds to the SNARE complex causing vesicle fusion and exocytosis. Mutations in *SYT2* (Whittaker et al. 2015), *VAMP1* (Salpietro et al. 2017), *SNAP25B* (Shen et al. 2014) and *MUNC13-1* cause presynaptic CMS.

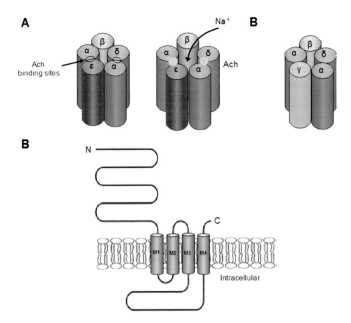

Figure 1.7   Schematic representation of the adult and fetal acetylcholine receptors. A The AChR is made up of five subunits arranged around a central pore. The binding of acetylcholine to the ACh binding sites results in a conformational change that allows the influx of sodium into the muscle and the trigger of an EPP. The fetal AChR has a γ-subunit (green) as opposed to the adult AChR, where the γ-subunit is replaced by an ε-subunit (red). **B** Each AChR subunit is composed of an extracellular domain, four transmembrane domains (M1–M4) and a large cytoplasmic loop that links M3 and M4. ACh, acetylcholine; AChR, acetylcholine receptor; EPP, endplate potential.

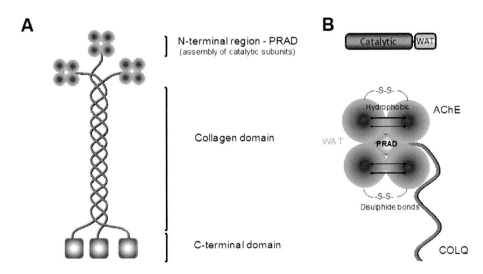

Figure 1.8   Schematic representation of acetylcholinesterase and its collagenic-like tail. A ColQ is composed of a N-terminal domain with a Proline Rich Attachment Domain (PRAD) that binds to the catalytic subunits of AChE, a triple-helix collagenic domain, and a C-terminal domain. **B** AChE is composed of a catalytic domain followed by a WAT (tryptophan [W] amphiphilic tetramerisation) domain at the C-terminal region. The association between catalytic subunits is primarily driven by the interaction between WAT domains (green colour) and PRAD (Chen et al. 2011). Additional forces include hydrophobic interactions and disulphide bonds. AChE, acetylcholinesterase.

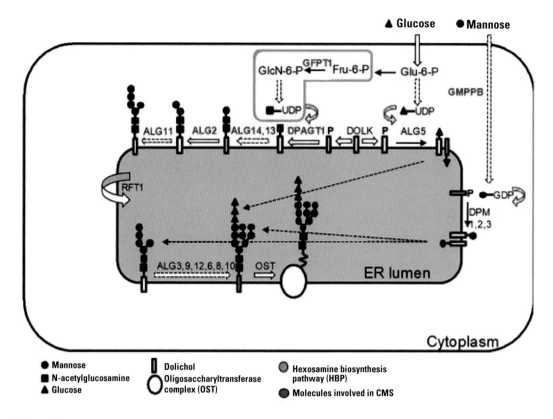

Figure 1.9 Simplified representation of the *N*-glycosylation pathway of proteins. The *N*-linked glycosylation of proteins takes place in the endoplasmic reticulum. It starts with the assembly of the core glycan (*N*-acetylglucosamine, glucose and mannose) on the lipid dolichol. A series of cytosolic glycosyltransferases proceed to dolichol glycosylation on the cytoplasmic face of the endoplasmic reticulum: GFPT1 synthesises UDP-GlcNAc (uridine diphosphate *N*-acetylglucosamine); DPAGT1 and the ALG13/14 complex are involved in adding the first and second *N*-acetylglucosamine to dolichol. Additional sugar residues are added by ALG2 and other enzymes until the resulting product is flipped into the endoplasmic reticulum lumen by RFT1. Inside the endoplasmic reticulum lumen, sugar moieties are incorporated until the glycan is transferred to asparagine residues of nascent proteins by the multimeric oligosaccharyl transferase complex (OST) that subsequently will be modified inside the endoplasmic reticulum and Golgi. DOLK, dolichol kinase; DPM, dolichol-phosphate mannose synthase; Fru-6-P, fructose-6-phosphate; GlcN-6-P, glucosamine-6-phosphate; Glu-6-P, glucose-6-phosphate; GMPPB, GDP-mannose pyrophosphorylase B. Adapted from Rodríguez Cruz (2016) with permission from BMJ Publishing Group Limited.

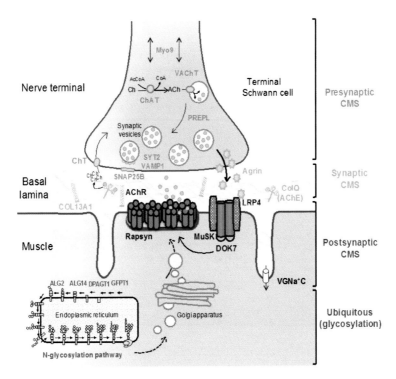

Figure 6.1   Schematic representation of the neuromuscular junction (NMJ) and the principle molecules involved in congenital myasthenia. The heterogeneous spectrum of mutated proteins and molecular mechanisms involved in congentical myasthenia syndromes (CMS) are illustrated. CMS results from presynaptic (ChAT, ChT, MUNC13-1, MYO9, PREPL, SYT2, VAChT, VAMP1), synaptic basal lamina abnormalities (COLQ, COL13A1) and postsynaptic defects (AChR subunits: α, β, δ and ε, AGRN, DOK7, MuSK, LRP4 and RAPSN). Additionally, the new genes encoding for molecules not confined to the NMJ (*GFPT1*, *DPAGT1*, *ALG2*, *ALG14* and *GMPPB*) are represented in the endoplasmic reticulum (ER), in a simplified view of the N-glycosylation pathway, together with the post-translational modifications of the saccharide structure of the AChR and other NMJ proteins inside the ER and Golgi apparatus, before reaching the muscle cell surface as mature proteins. ACh, acetylcholine; AChE, acetylcholinesterase; AcCoA, acetyl coenzyme A; AChR, acetylcholine receptor; Ch, choline; VGNa⁺C, voltage-gated sodium channel. Reproduced from Rodríguez Cruz et al. (2018) with permission.

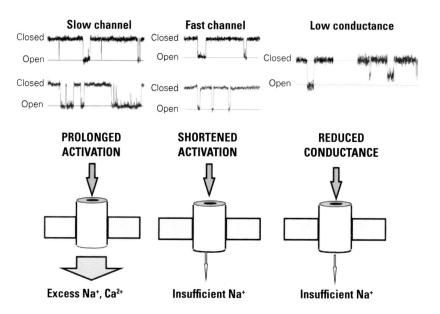

Figure 6.2 **Illustration of the pathogenic mechanisms of disorders of the acetylcholine receptor ion channel.** Top panels illustrate patch clamp single acetylcholine receptor channel recording traces: black traces, wild-type channels; red traces, mutant channels. Lower panels illustrate the consequence of altered ion channel function. Reproduced from Beeson (2012) with permission from Wiley.

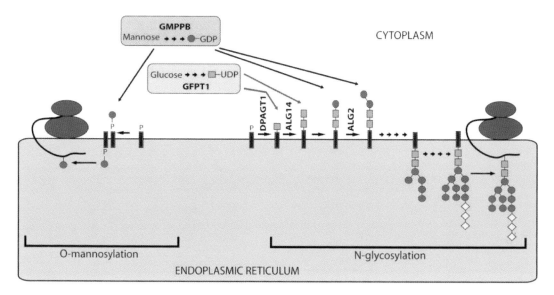

Figure 6.3 **Simplified scheme of N-linked and O-linked glycosylation showing the five glycosylation genes *(GFPT1, DPAGT1, ALG2, ALG14 and GMPPB)*** associated with the congenital myasthenia syndromes. Reproduced from Belaya et al. (2015) with permission from Oxford University Press.

led to subjective improvement and quantitatively better-timed tests of function. Effect was sustained at 6 months. Another 7-year-old boy with a *TPM3* mutation was born at term with low tone and feeding issues. He walked at 14 months but could not run or jump and had respiratory infections. Facial weakness with ptosis and fatigability persisted as he grew older. Muscle biopsy revealed type 1 fibre hypotrophy. Stimulated SFEMG showed increased jitter; pyridostigmine was offered but declined by his guardian.

Ryanodine Receptor 1 Mutations

Ryanodine receptor-1 (RYR1) has a role in calcium release which in turn is important in excitation-contraction coupling of skeletal muscle. Clinically diverse presentations have been seen with *RYR1* mutations. Two cases of siblings with *RYR1* mutations were described (Illingworth et al. 2014). The older brother presented with low tone, fluctuating ptosis, with a course that included loss of tone during crawling, bulbar weakness and ophthalmoplegia. A pyridostigmine trial (7mg/kg/day) at 3 years of age was reported to improve facial expression, ptosis and stamina per parents. Episodes of hypotonia resolved and his voice was louder. Ambulation declined with increasing reliability on wheelchair use between 4 and 7 years of age. Addition of salbutamol at 2mg three times daily enabled ambulation with use of a walker. The child's younger sister was similar but milder in presentation. She was started on a pyridostigmine trial at 18 months of age with improvement in facial expression and stamina. Muscle biopsy featured type 1 fibre hypotrophy suggestive of CFTD. EMG and SFEMG which were only possible at ages 7 and 5, respectively, showed a myopathic phenotype without increased jitter. Genetic testing for the siblings showed two heterozygous mutations in *RYR1* and parental testing revealed heterozygous carrier status with mother carrying one mutation and father the other.

Cap Myopathies

Cap myopathy involves most muscles, but muscles of the face, neck, and limbs are most severely affected. Muscle biopsy demonstrates cap-like structures consisting of disorganised myofibrils with Z lines (Goebel 2007). Severity of myopathy correlates with percentage of muscle cells displaying these abnormal caps. Cap myopathy has been described with mutations in the *ACTA1*, tropomyosin 2 (*TPM2*) or *TPM3* genes (Clarke et al. 2009; De Paula et al. 2009; Hung et al. 2010). Cases are autosomal dominant or de novo. A 16-year-old male was described with cap myopathy and NMT defect (Rodríguez Cruz et al. 2014). At birth, this male infant was noted to have ptosis, facial weakness and poor feeding. With the presence of fluctuation in symptoms noted at 2 months of age, a pyridostigmine trial was initiated resulting in improvement of spontaneous movements, facial weakness and feeding. The tensilon test of ACEI was positive and by age 7 years he was able to climb stairs. Speech fatigue persisted, and he needed nocturnal NIV for hypoventilation. At 12 years of age SFEMG was normal and RNS was refused. Muscle biopsy showed features suggestive of caps. Sequencing was positive for a heterozygous deletion in exon 4 of the tropomyosin 2 (*TPM2*) gene. Pyridostigmine at 45mg four times daily was continued with good response.

CONCLUSIONS

Historically, early onset of ptosis, ophthalmoparesis and other features of fatigability have been thought to mostly suggest a congenital myasthenic syndrome. With more causative genes being discovered in neuromuscular disorders, possible roles of these in the NMJ structure and maintenance is emerging. Table 8.1 summarizes the various neuromuscular disorders with defects in neuromuscular transmission and lists the

Table 8.1   Neuromuscular disorders with genes reported to have transmission defects

Disorder	Genes
Anterior horn diseases	
Spinal muscular atrophy	SMN
Spinal and bulbar muscular atrophy	AR
Myotonic dystrophy	DMPK
Congenital muscular dystrophy	LARGE
Duchenne muscular dystrophy	Dystrophin
Congenital disorders of glycosylation	DPAGT1, GFPT1, ALG2, ALG14
Congenital myopathies	
Nemaline myopathy	KLHL40
Centronuclear myopathy	MTM1, DNM2, BIN1
Congenital fibre type disproportion	TPM3, RYR1
Cap disease	TPM2
Mitochondrial	SLC25A1
Other	LAMA5, PLECTIN

associated genes. As illustrated in this chapter, multiple authors have shown neuromuscular transmission defects in both animal models and clinical human disease that do not have primary pathology in the neuromuscular junction. It is interesting and clinically useful to note that these illustrative models and individuals have had improvement in fatigue with the use of ACEIs and/or other modulators of neuromuscular transmission (ephedrine, 3,4-DAP, salbutamol). To conclude, multiple neuromuscular disorders should be considered in the differential diagnosis when children present with symptoms and signs of neuromuscular transmission defects. Conversely, myasthenic syndromes ought to be in the differential deliberations of a myopathic phenotype. Furthermore, the use of medications that improve neuromuscular transmission should be considered in their symptomatic treatment.

REFERENCES

Aminoff MJ, Layzer RB, Satya-Murti S, Faden AI (1977) The declining electrical response of muscle to repetitive nerve stimulation in myotonia. *Neurology* **27:** 812–816.

Armstrong GA, Drapeau P (2013) Loss and gain of FUS function impair neuromuscular synaptic transmission in a genetic model of ALS. *Hum Mol Genet* **22:** 4282–4292.

Arnold AS, Gueye M, Guettier-Sigrist S et al. (2004) Reduced expression of nicotinic AChRs in myotubes from spinal muscular atrophy I patients. *Lab Invest* **84:** 1271–1278.

Benoit P, Changeux JP (1975) Consequences of tenotomy on the evolution of multiinnervation in developing rat soleus muscle. *Brain Res* **99:** 354–358.

Bird TD (1993) Myotonic dystrophy type 1. In: Adam MP, Ardinger HH, Pagon RA, Wallace SE, Bean LJH, Stephens K et al. (Eds), *GeneReviews®*. Seattle, WA.

Birnkrant DJ, Bushby K, Bann CM et al. (2018) Diagnosis and management of Duchenne muscular dystrophy, part 1: diagnosis, and neuromuscular, rehabilitation, endocrine, and gastroin- testinal and nutritional management. *Lancet Neurol* **17:** 251–267.

Blake DJ, Weir A, Newey SE, Davies KE (2002) Function and genetics of dystrophin and dystrophin-related proteins in muscle. *Physiol Rev* **82**: 291–329.

Bombelli F, Lispi L, Porrini SC et al. (2016) Neuromuscular trans- mission abnormalities in myotonic dystrophy type 1: A neurophysiological study. *Clin Neurol Neurosurg* **150**: 84–88.

Bowerman M, Murray LM, Beauvais A, Pinheiro B, Kothary R (2012) A critical smn threshold in mice dictates onset of an intermediate spinal muscular atrophy phenotype associated with a distinct neuromuscular junction pathology. *Neuromuscul Disord* **22**: 263–276.

Brady S, Morfini G (2010) A perspective on neuronal cell death signaling and neurodegeneration. *Mol Neurobiol* **42**: 25–31.

Brenner HR, Lømo T, Williamson R (1987) Control of end-plate channel properties by neurotrophic effects and by muscle activity in rat. *J Physiol* **388**: 367–381.

Cassandrini D, Trovato R, Rubegni A et al. (2017) Congenital myopathies: clinical phenotypes and new diagnostic tools. *Ital J Pediatr* **43**: 101.

Chand KK, Lee KM, Lee JD et al. (2018) Defects in synaptic transmission at the neuromuscular junction precede motor deficits in a TDP-43Q331K transgenic mouse model of amyotrophic lateral sclerosis. *FASEB J* **32**: 2676–2689.

Chaouch A, Porcelli V, Cox D et al. (2014) Mutations in the mitochondrial citrate carrier SLC25A1 are associated with impaired neuromuscular transmission. *J Neuromuscul Dis* **1**: 75–90.

Claeys KG, Maisonobe T, Böhm J et al. (2010) Phenotype of a patient with recessive centronuclear myopathy and a novel BIN1 mutation. *Neurology* **74**: 519–521.

Clarke NF, Domazetovska A, Waddell L, Kornberg A, McLean C, North KN (2009) Cap disease due to mutation of the beta-tropomyosin gene (TPM2). *Neuromuscul Disord* **19**: 348–351.

Clarke NF, North KN (2003) Congenital fiber type disproportion—30 years on. *J Neuropathol Exp Neurol* **62(10)**: 977–989.

De Paula AM, Franques J, Fernandez C et al. (2009) A TPM3 mutation causing cap myopathy. *Neuromuscul Disord* **19**: 685–688.

Deconinck AE, Rafael JA, Skinner JA et al. (1997) Utrophin-dystrophin- deficient mice as a model for Duchenne muscular dystrophy. *Cell* **90**: 717–727.

Edvardson S, Porcelli V, Jalas C et al. (2013) Agenesis of corpus callosum and optic nerve hypoplasia due to mutations in SLC25A1 encoding the mitochondrial citrate transporter. *J Med Genet* **50**: 240–245.

Elder GB, Dean D, McComas AJ, Paes B, DeSa D (1983) Infantile centronuclear myopathy. Evidence suggesting incomplete innervation. *J Neurol Sci* **60**: 79–88.

Fahim MA (1989) Rapid neuromuscular remodeling following limb immobilization. *Anat Rec* **224**: 102–109.

Fan L, Simard LR (2002) Survival motor neuron (SMN) protein: role in neurite outgrowth and neuromuscular maturation during neuronal differentiation and development. *Hum Mol Genet* **11**: 1605–1614.

Ferri A, Sanes JR, Coleman MP, Cunningham JM, Kato AC (2003) Inhibiting axon degeneration and synapse loss attenuates apoptosis and disease progression in a mouse model of motoneuron disease. *Curr Biol* **13**: 669–673.

Fidziańska A (1980) Human ontogenesis. II. Development of the human neuromuscular junction. *J Neuropathol Exp Neurol* **39**: 606–615.

Fidziańska A, Goebel HH (1994) Aberrant arrested in maturation neuromuscular junctions in centronuclear myopathy. *J Neurol Sci* **124**: 83–88.

Frey D, Schneider C, Xu L, Borg J, Spooren W, Caroni P (2000) Early and selective loss of neuromuscular synapse subtypes with low sprouting competence in motoneuron diseases. *J Neurosci* **20**: 2534–2542.

Gibbs EM, Clarke NF, Rose K et al. (2013) Neuromuscular junction abnormalities in DNM2-related centronuclear myopathy. *J Mol Med (Berl)* **91**: 727–737.

Goebel HH (2007) Cap disease uncapped. *Neuromuscul Disord* **17**: 429–432.

Grady RM, Teng H, Nichol MC, Cunningham JC, Wilkinson RS, Sanes JR (1997) Skeletal and cardiac myopathies in mice lacking utrophin and dystrophin: a model for Duchenne muscular dystrophy. *Cell* **90**: 729–738.

Herman GE, Kopacz K, Zhao W, Mills PL, Metzenberg A, Das S (2002) Characterization of mutations in fifty North American patients with X-linked myotubular myopathy. *Hum Mutat* **19**: 114–121.

Hung RM, Yoon G, Hawkins CE, Halliday W, Biggar D, Vajsar J (2010) Cap myopathy caused by a mutation of the skeletal alpha-actin gene ACTA1. *Neuromuscul Disord* **20:** 238–240.

Illingworth MA, Main M, Pitt M et al. (2014) RYR1-related congenital myopathy with fatigable weakness, responding to pyridostigimine. *Neuromuscul Disord* **24:** 707–712.

Iwanami T, Sonoo M, Hatanaka Y, Hokkoku K, Oishi C, Shimizu T (2011) Decremental responses to repetitive nerve stimulation (RNS) in motor neuron disease. *Clin Neurophysiol* **122:** 2530–2536.

Jungbluth H, Wallgren-Pettersson C, Laporte J (2008) Centronuclear (myotubular) myopathy. *Orphanet J Rare Dis* **3:** 26.

Kariya S, Park GH, Maeno-Hikichi Y et al. (2008) Reduced SMN protein impairs maturation of the neuromuscular junctions in mouse models of spinal muscular atrophy. *Hum Mol Genet* **17:** 2552–2569.

Katsuno M, Adachi H, Minamiyama M et al. (2006) Reversible disruption of dynactin 1-mediated retrograde axonal transport in polyglutamine-induced motor neuron degeneration. *J Neurosci* **26:** 12106–12117.

Kawase K, Nishino I, Sugimoto M et al. (2015) Nemaline myopathy with KLHL40 mutation presenting as congenital totally locked-in state. *Brain Dev* **37:** 887–890.

Kemp MQ, Poort JL, Baqri RM et al. (2011) Impaired motoneuronal retro- grade transport in two models of SBMA implicates two sites of androgen action. *Hum Mol Genet* **20:** 4475–4490.

Killian JM, Wilfong AA, Burnett L, Appel SH, Boland D (1994) Decremental motor responses to repetitive nerve stimulation in ALS. *Muscle Nerve* **17:** 747–754.

Kim JY, Park KD, Kim SM, Sunwoo IN (2011) Repetitive nerve stimulation test in amyotrophic lateral sclerosis with predominant oropharyngeal manifestations. *J Clin Neurol* **7:** 31–33.

Kolb SJ, Kissel JT (2011) Spinal muscular atrophy: a timely review. *Arch Neurol* **68:** 979–984.

Kong L, Wang X, Choe DW et al. (2009) Impaired synaptic vesicle release and immaturity of neuromuscular junctions in spinal muscular atrophy mice. *J Neurosci* **29:** 842–851.

Kress W, Rost S, Kolokotronis K, Meng G, Pluta N, Müller-Reible C (2017) The genetic approach: Next-generation sequencing-based diagnosis of congenital and infantile myopathies/muscle dystrophies. *Neuropediatrics* **48:** 242–246.

Krishnan AV, Kiernan MC (2006) Axonal function and activity-dependent excitability changes in myotonic dystrophy. *Muscle Nerve* **33(5):** 627–636.

Liewluck T, Shen XM, Milone M, Engel AG (2011) Endplate structure and parameters of neuromuscular transmission in sporadic centronuclear myopathy associated with myasthenia. *Neuromuscul Disord* **21:** 387–395.

Lin TL, Chen TH, Hsu YY, Cheng YH, Juang BT, Jong YJ (2016) Selective neuromuscular denervation in Taiwanese severe SMA mouse can be reversed by morpholino antisense oligonucleotides. *PLoS One* **11:** e0154723.

Ling KK, Gibbs RM, Feng Z, Ko CP (2012) Severe neuromuscular denervation of clinically relevant muscles in a mouse model of spinal muscular atrophy. *Hum Mol Genet* **21:** 185–195.

Lunn MR, Wang CH (2008) Spinal muscular atrophy. *Lancet* **371:** 2120–2133.

MacDermot V (1961) The histology of the neuromuscular junction in dystrophia myotonica. *Brain* **84:** 75–84.

McFarland R, Taylor RW, Turnbull DM (2010) A neurological perspective on mitochondrial disease. *Lancet Neurol* **9:** 829–840.

Munot P, Lashley D, Jungbluth H, Feng L, Pitt M, Robb SA et al. (2010) Congenital fibre type disproportion associated with mutations in the tropomyosin 3 (TPM3) gene mimicking congenital myasthenia. *Neuromuscul Disord* **20:** 796–800.

Murray LM, Comley LH, Thomson D, Parkinson N, Talbot K, Gillingwater TH (2008) Selective vulnerability of motor neurons and dissociation of pre- and post-synaptic pathology at the neuromuscular junction in mouse models of spinal muscular atrophy. *Hum Mol Genet* **17:** 949–962.

Natera-de Benito D, Nascimento A, Abicht A et al. (2016) KLHL40-related nemaline myopathy with a sustained, positive response to treatment with acetylcholinesterase inhibitors. *J Neurol* **263:** 517–523.

North KN (2011) Clinical approach to the diagnosis of congenital myopathies. *Semin Pediatr Neurol* **18:** 216–220.

Panaite PA, Gantelet E, Kraftsik R, Gourdon G, Kuntzer T, Barakat-Walter I (2008) Myotonic dystrophy transgenic mice exhibit pathologic abnormalities in diaphragm neuromuscular junctions and phrenic nerves. *J Neuropathol Exp Neurol* **67:** 763–772.

Preterre C, Magot A, Geneau Bodis F et al. (2015) Repetitive nerve stimulation in spinal muscular atrophy. *Neuromuscul Disord* **25:** S194.

Ravenscroft G, Miyatake S, Lehtokari VL et al. (2013) Mutations in KLHL40 are a frequent cause of severe autosomal-recessive nemaline myopathy. *Am J Hum Genet* **93:** 6–18.

Robb SA, Sewry CA, Dowling JJ et al. (2011) Impaired neuromuscular transmission and response to acetylcholinesterase inhibitors in centronuclear myopathies. *Neuromuscul Disord* **21:** 379–386.

Rocha MC, Pousinha PA, Correia AM, Sebastião AM, Ribeiro JA (2013) Early changes of neuromuscular transmission in the SOD1(G93A) mice model of ALS start long before motor symptoms onset. *PLoS One* **8:** e73846.

Rodríguez Cruz PM, Sewry C, Beeson D et al. (2014) Congenital myopathies with secondary neuromuscular transmission defects; a case report and review of the literature. *Neuromuscul Disord* **24:** 1103–1110.

Romero NB (2010) Centronuclear myopathies: a widening concept. *Neuromuscul Disord* **20:** 223–228.

Sewry CA (2008) Pathological defects in congnital myopathies. *J Muscle Res Cell Motil* **29(6–8):** 2311–2238.

Shahidullah M, Le Marchand SJ, Fei H et al. (2013) Defects in synapse structure and function precede motor neuron degeneration in Drosophila models of FUS-related ALS. *J Neurosci* **33:** 19590–19598.

Thompson W, Kuffler DP, Jansen JK (1979) The effect of prolonged, reversible block of nerve impulses on the elimination of polyneuronal innervation of new-born rat skeletal muscle fibers. *Neuroscience* **4:** 271–281.

van der Pijl EM, van Putten M, Niks EH, Verschuuren JJ, Aartsma-Rus A, Plomp JJ (2016) Characterization of neuromuscular synapse function abnormalities in multiple Duchenne muscular dystrophy mouse models. *Eur J Neurosci* **43(12):** 1623–1635.

Wadman RI, Vrancken AF, van den Berg LH, van der Pol WL (2012) Dysfunction of the neuromuscular junction in spinal muscular atrophy types 2 and 3. *Neurology* **79:** 2050–2055.

Wallgren-Pettersson C, Sewry CA, Nowak KJ, Laing NG (2011) Nemaline myopathies. *Semin Pediatr Neurol* **18:** 230–238.

Wheeler TM, Krym MC, Thornton CA (2007) Ribonuclear foci at the neuromuscular junction in myotonic dystrophy type 1. *Neuromuscul Disord* **17:** 242–247.

Wood SJ, Slater CR (2001) Safety factor at the neuromuscular junction. *Prog Neurobiol* **64:** 393–429.

Xu Y, Halievski K, Henley C et al. (2016) Defects in neuromuscular transmission may underlie motor dysfunction in spinal and bulbar muscular atrophy. *J Neurosci* **36:** 5094–5106.

Respiratory Care in Childhood Myasthenia

Andrew Ives

Fatigable muscle weakness that is the cardinal feature of myasthenia can have major repercussions for the respiratory system, primarily through its effects on the following muscle groups:

- Respiratory muscles – especially the diaphragm and intercostals. Weakness here will directly affect breathing.
- Muscles of bulbar function – affecting swallowing and feeding. Weakness can cause pooling of secretions and ineffective sucking/swallowing, with the associated risk of aspiration and lung injury.

TRANSIENT NEONATAL MYASTHENIA

Transient neonatal myasthenia caused by transplacental transfer of maternal antibodies can cause severe respiratory difficulties in the newborn period. Estimates of rates of neonatal myasthenia range from 5% to 30% of infants born to mothers with autoimmune myasthenia gravis (Papazian 1992; Jovandaric et al. 2016; Peragallo 2017). Around one-third of pregnancies in mothers with myasthenia gravis end with a premature delivery (Jovandaric et al. 2016), with the associated risk of respiratory complications that premature delivery carries. There is no good correlation between maternal disease and neonatal disease severity (Jovandaric et al. 2016). Most mothers of affected infants do have active disease, but some may be in remission (Elias et al. 1979) or have no signs of disease (Verspyck et al. 1993). Occasionally the infant's symptoms lead to a maternal diagnosis (Papazian 1992).

Symptoms

Approximately two-thirds of affected children have onset of symptoms within a few hours of birth; nearly 80% present within 24 hours (Papazian 1992). Onset after the third day of life is rare (Papazian 1992; Jovandaric et al. 2016).

The most common presenting symptoms are (Hutchison and Russell 1979):

- poor cry;
- poor suck and swallow (and pooling of secretions);
- feeding difficulty (including fatigability during feeds);
- generalised weakness;
- respiratory difficulty – varying from mild tachypnoea to severe distress requiring mechanical ventilation.

Treatment

All babies born to mothers known to have myasthenia gravis (even if the mother's disease is well controlled) should be examined and observed for evidence of transient myasthenic weakness for 3–5 days (Sanders et al. 2016).

Around 80% of patients need some form of supportive management. Respiratory distress needing ventilation is seen in nearly one-third of cases (Papazian), although the duration of ventilation is not normally prolonged. Bulbar dysfunction may require support such as nasogastric tube feeding.

Symptoms are self-limiting and the weakness improves as the maternal antibodies are cleared from the infant circulation. Full recovery is seen in 90% of babies within 2 months and by 4 months in all (Papazian 1992).

AUTOIMMUNE MYASTHENIA

The respiratory compromise seen in autoimmune myasthenia is well described; weakness and respiratory insufficiency were also part of the first animal model of autoimmune myasthenia developed by Lindstrom et al. (1976), in which rats that were injected with highly purified acetylcholine receptor (AChR) antibodies developed respiratory insufficiency within 3 weeks.

Respiratory Muscle Weakness in Autoimmune Myasthenia

Respiratory muscle weakness in most neuromuscular diseases usually occurs in the context of severe and diffuse muscle weakness and occurs relatively late in the disease. Respiratory failure early in the course of the disease process can occur more rarely and can occur in autoimmune myasthenia, where it is one of the most common diseases with this presentation (Pfeffer et al. 2015). Respiratory difficulty can be especially pronounced when there is diaphragmatic muscle weakness.

In one case series, 10% of patients had respiratory failure as their initial disease presentation (Qureshi et al. 2004). A review of studies by Chiang et al. (2009) found that, across nine studies, from 2% to 50% of primarily paediatric patients have symptoms at first presentation of Osserman grade 3 or 4 – moderate or severe generalised weakness, bulbar dysfunction or both. Overall 12% (89/717) of patients presented with this severity that would very likely have some respiratory manifestations. Postpubertal patients seem more likely to present with generalised symptoms when compared to prepubertal children; this variability seems to some degree to be ethnically based with Asian children more likely to have an ocular presentation. A range of 29–75% of patients have generalised disease, either at presentation or later, with the lower percentages reported in the more recent studies. Juvenile autoimmune myasthenia can also present as recurrent pulmonary infection and atelectasis (Unal et al. 2007).

Patients who are muscle-specific kinase (MuSK) antibody positive can have a more severe form of the disease with a greater risk of respiratory compromise and more pronounced bulbar signs (Evoli et al. 2003; Sanders et al. 2003; Gadient et al. 2009).

Bulbar Symptoms in Autoimmune Myasthenia

Around 15% of patients present with bulbar symptoms due to oropharyngeal muscular weakness. This may just be fatigable chewing, but there can also be difficulty swallowing and choking when eating and drinking. This carries a risk of aspiration and its associated potential for causing lung disease. Bulbar weakness can affect up to 75% of patients at some point (Gadient et al. 2009). Bulbar weakness can be profound during a crisis, and increasing bulbar symptoms should be taken as an important warning sign.

The Myasthenic Crisis

The most serious and important respiratory manifestation of autoimmune myasthenia is the myasthenic crisis, where respiratory muscle involvement causes respiratory insufficiency and failure. The International Consensus Guidance for Management of Myasthenia Gravis definines a myasthenic crisis as a "worsening of myasthenic weakness requiring intubation or noninvasive ventilation, except when these measures are employed during routine postoperative management" (Sanders et al. 2016). Ventilatory failure (with no peripheral neuromuscular involvement) may be the only clinically overt manifestation of a crisis (Dushay et al. 1990). Respiratory failure in autoimmune myasthenia is associated with 10% mortality during or immediately after the episode and can lead to prolonged intensive care admission (Thomas et al. 1997).

Most crises occur in the first few years after diagnosis when the disease is in its most active phase. Already weak respiratory muscles can fatigue suddenly, precipitating a respiratory collapse. Crises can be precipitated by surgery, infections, pregnancy, some drugs (for example antibiotics) or a reduction of immunosuppressive treatment. There may be no clear trigger with the crisis occurring during an active phase of the disease as part of the normal natural history. Thymectomy, performed as part of disease therapy, can also precipitate a crisis. This can be relatively common, occurring in over 10% of patients in one study (Watanabe et al. 2004). In this study higher pre-operative levels of anti-AChR antibody (>100nmol/L) and large operative blood loss (>1L) were independent predictors of post-op crises. Crises may be more common in younger children; a Norwegian study found that 21% of prepubertal children had myasthenic crises requiring respiratory assistance compared with 5% of postpubertal children (Popperud et al. 2017).

Respiratory Drugs and the Myasthenic Crisis

Many drugs are known to precipitate myasthenic crises. Some drugs are particularly likely to be used in respiratory disease and so these must be used with caution in patients with myasthenia.

Corticosteroids (e.g. prednisolone) are a common treatment in myasthenia. Their ability to cause myopathy is, however, well known (Schakman et al. 2008) and at high doses they may cause a significant exacerbation of myasthenia symptoms during the early stages of treatment. For this reason, glucocorticoids, especially if given in high doses, should only be used in patients in hospital where intravenous immunoglobulin (IVIG) or plasmapheresis may be used to manage any acute deterioration (Richman and Agius 2003).

Superimposed infections in myasthenic patients can increase morbidity and mortality, particularly as they can precipitate a crisis. Infections therefore must be aggressively treated, but antibiotics must be chosen carefully as many have been associated with the worsening of myasthenic symptoms (Table 9.1). Fluoroquinolones, aminoglycosides and macrolides seem to be the most high risk.

Sleep in Autoimmune Myasthenia

In typically developing children, in sleep, upper airway resistance increases, chemosensitivity is reduced and the wakefulness drive to breathe is lost, resulting in a fall in ventilation (Bourke and Gibson 2002).

In patients with respiratory muscle weakness, sleep is fragmented with a shorter total sleep time, frequent arousals and a reduction in rapid eye movement (REM) sleep. Sleep disordered breathing and nocturnal desaturations are common (especially if there is diaphragmatic weakness) and are most severe during the remaining REM sleep (Quera-Salva et al. 1992). In adults, abnormalities can be seen even in those with mild myasthenia (Manni et al. 1995) and overall sleep disordered breathing is common in myasthenia, and can be severe enough to mimic a crisis (Lai et al. 2016). These issues may improve after

Table 9.1   Antibiotics that can worsen myasthenic weakness

Antibiotic	Notes	Reference
Macrolides	Esp. Telithromycin	Jennett et al. (2006)
Fluoroquinolones	Esp. Ciprofloxacin; moxifloxacin; levofloxacin	Jones et al. (2011)
Aminoglycosides		Barrons (1997)
Penicillins	E.g. Ampicillin	Argov et al. (1986)
Polymixins	E.g. Colistimethate	McQuillen et al. (1968)
Carbapenems	E.g. Imipinem/cilastatin	O'Riordan et al. (1994)
Lincosamides	Clindamycin has been reported to cause neuromuscular blockade	al Ahdal and Bevan (1995)

thymectomy (Amino et al. 1998) or with immune modulation. Night-time bilevel positive airways pressure (BiPAP) should be started if there is significant nocturnal hypoventilation. Some patients may also need it in the day for rest periods.

Respiratory Investigations

All patients with autoimmune myasthenia, particularly those at risk of a crisis, should have regular assessments of respiratory function which should include observation of important clinical signs (Table 9.2). The generalised weakness that can be present can sometimes mask the usual signs of respiratory distress such as accessory muscle use; in these cases more subtle signs, such as tachycardia, need to be observed for.

Many patients with autoimmune myasthenia have evidence of reduced respiratory muscle strength as measured by maximum inspiratory and expiratory pressure (MIP and MEP) (Keenan et al. 1995). They can also have a reduced forced expiratory volume in 1 second (FEV1) and forced vital capacity (FVC) in a restrictive pattern (Griggs et al. 1981). These measures, and oxygen saturations, should also be measured several times a day for patients at risk. Low oxygen saturations indicate alveolar hypoventilation which is an important indicator of impending respiratory failure. If weakness progresses then ultimately fatigue, hypercarbia and ventilatory insufficiency occur.

These investigations can show abnormalities even if there is no respiratory distress but they can also be maintained even after the (sometimes sudden) onset of respiratory failure. Pulmonary function tests may therefore be poorly predictive of the need for mechanical ventilation (Rieder et al. 1995).

Overnight sleep studies should be performed if there is a concern about significant nocturnal hypoventilation.

Table 9.2   Important clinical signs in myasthenia (indicating respiratory distress, failure or hypoxia)

Dyspnoea (especially when lying supine)
Weak cough
Dysphagia
Pooling of/inability to clear secretions
Hypophonia
Increased (or decreased) respiratory effort
Tachycardia
Restlessness
Agitation
Insomnia

Respiratory Management

Cholinesterase inhibitors used in the pharmacotherapy of myasthenia gravis can have profound muscarinic side effects, including increased airway secretions. This can worsen breathing problems and so these drugs often need to be used in combination with antimuscarinic drugs such as hyoscine (generally given as transdermal patches) or glycopyrrolate.

Myasthenic crises require aggressive management and supportive care, usually in a high dependency or intensive care unit. Intensive care and mechanical vent may also be needed as postoperative support after thymectomy. Respiratory function should therefore be maximised prior to thymectomy by optimal treatment of the underlying myasthenia; steroids can be very effective at preventing respiratory insufficiency in this situation (Kataoka et al. 2014). Severe crises may require ventilatory support, which in its various forms can be needed for several days to a few weeks (Piastra et al. 2005). Noninvasive ventilation (NIV) can be tried initially, before severe hypoventilation occurs, where its use can prevent the need for invasive ventilation while the patient improves due to pharmacotherapy, IVIG or plasma exchange. It can also help to avert sedation, intubation and the complications of invasive ventilation (Rabinstein and Wijdicks 2002; Rabinstein 2005; Seneviratne et al. 2008a). It can be well tolerated, even in children, but the face mask interface can be poorly tolerated and can cause problems in those with weak cough, severe bulbar dysfunction and/or copious respiratory secretions. Some patients with bulbar symptoms can tolerate it well however (Rabinstein 2005).

There are no good criteria for who should start on NIV and who should be intubated immediately. Studies in adults suggest that a pCO_2 of more than 45mmHg (Seneviratne et al. 2008a) or more than 50mmHg (Rabinstein and Wijdicks 2002) on NIV initiation predicts the need for later intubation. Patients in whom NIV has failed often develop pneumonia and atelectasis (Thomas et al. 1997). This can be minimised by the use of physiotherapy, airway secretion suctioning, antibiotics, and bronchodilators (Varelas et al. 2002). Invasive ventilation may be required if the patient's clinical condition is particularly severe or NIV has failed. It has the advantage of offering more aggressive respiratory support as well as better airway protection and secretion clearance.

Weaning and extubation can only be tried once secretions are controlled and once muscle strength is improving (aided by optimal myasthenia drug therapy). Extubation failure occurs in nearly half of patients (Seneviratne et al. 2008b) and reintubation is needed in approximately one-quarter (Rabinstein 2005; Seneviratne et al. 2008b). The presence of atelectasis has a strong association with both; failed extubation is otherwise associated with prolonged ventilation, male sex, older age and previous crises (Rabinstein 2005; Seneviratne et al. 2008b). The need for reintubation is also predicted by low vital capacity and the need for BiPAP after extubation (although NIV can be used to allow a patient to transition off invasive ventilation); younger patients also tended to have a greater risk. Respiratory physiotherapy during periods of weakness or respiratory support is therefore vital to aid secretion clearance and to treat any atelectasis. Effective coughing is essential for the removal of airway secretions and a weak or ineffective cough predisposes patients to atelectasis, aspiration and chest infections. Airway suctioning and cough assist devices may therefore be helpful. Failure to wean a patient off invasive ventilation may mean that tracheostomy insertion is required.

Other Issues

All patients should have a regularly updated respiratory care plan in the event of deterioration.

Patients should be fully immunised according to the relevant national schedule. This should include pneumococcal vaccination and the seasonal influenza vaccine. Several studies have shown the inactivated (intramuscular) influenza vaccine to be safe in myasthenic patients (Seok et al. 2017; Tackenberg et al.

2018). More caution needs to be taken with the live attenuated (nasal) influenza vaccine, especially for those patients on oral corticosteroids.

CONGENITAL MYASTHENIC SYNDROMES

Congenital myasthenic syndromes usually present in the first year of life (Palace et al. 2012) with fluctuating fatigable weakness affecting any of several muscle groups; as with other forms of myasthenia the respiratory and bulbar muscles are commonly affected and can be significantly so. There are often respiratory symptoms in the neonatal period (Kinali et al. 2008) and these early neonatal-onset forms can mimic transient neonatal myasthenia and lead to early respiratory failure and apnoea.

The severity of the congenital myasthenic syndromes is highly variable. Depending on the gene mutation, there is considerable phenotypic variation between the different forms of congenital myasthenia; this is also true with respect to the degree that the respiratory system is involved. There are often spontaneous bouts of the disease, commonly triggered by respiratory infections. Gastro-intestinal symptoms such as diarrhoea and vomiting can also cause fluctuations in muscle strength as myasthenia medication may be poorly absorbed (Robb et al. 2010).

At its worst the respiratory manifestations can include life-threatening apnoeas and respiratory distress or, in older children, a rapid progression from mild weakness to respiratory failure over the course of a few hours – in these forms the risk of death is high in the absence of medical help. There is overlap between the clinical features of different forms of congenital myasthenia and while hypoventilation can occur in all types of CMS, some forms are particularly prone to respiratory problems.

Fast-channel Syndrome

Fast-channel syndrome is usually the most severe form of CMS (Finlayson 2013b), with life-threatening respiratory crises in early infancy and childhood (Palace et al. 2012) on a background of severe generalised hypotonia and weakness. Episodic apnoeas and chronic hypoventilation require regular respiratory assessment and often home NIV (Finlayson 2013b). Patients are also affected from birth with bulbar/feeding problems leading to a risk of aspiration. Feeding problems continue into childhood and often require nasogastric feeding or gastrostomy.

DOK7 Mutations

Although DOK7 CMS usually presents in childhood with walking difficulties, up to one-third of patients have onset at birth with hypotonia, feeding problems and respiratory distress. The early-onset breathing difficulties can be severe enough to require respiratory support (Müller et al. 2007). Motor and respiratory degradation has been reported in later adulthood in patients who had initially only mild disease (Eymard et al. 2013), leading to progressive respiratory failure (Robb et al. 2010). Overall, around 70% of patients have respiratory involvement that varies from a mildly decreased FVC to severe problems needing ventilation. Fluctuations of weakness are common and can last weeks or months (Eymard et al. 2013). Overall, around 25% of patients require NIV at some point (Rodríguez Cruz et al. 2014). As with other forms of CMS, feeding difficulties can require support with nasogastric tube feeding or also occasionally gastrostomy tube insertion. A particular feature of *DOK7* mutations is the presence of early-onset stridor due to vocal cord palsy (Anderson et al. 2008; Ben Ammar et al. 2010). This can occur without significant weakness elsewhere and can be severe enough to require tracheostomy insertion. Congenital stridor and vocal cord palsy has also been reported in infants with other CMS mutations such as *RAPSYN* (Beri et al. 2009).

RAPSYN Congenital Myasthenia Syndrome

Patients with *RAPSYN* mutations frequently present with respiratory weakness at birth together with feeding problems and generalised hypotonia (Finlayson 2013b). Most patients present in the first year of life (Burke et al. 2003) and periods of mechanical ventilation are not unusual. Some have a milder form where there is a beginning in childhood or even adulthood (Eymard et al. 2013).

Acute life-threatening crises with respiratory failure and bulbar symptoms are frequent, particularly during infancy and early childhood. Crises usually (but not always) occur in the context of infections and can be severe enough to cause anoxic encephalopathy (Engel et al. 2015). Severe respiratory difficulties have been reported after general anaesthesia (Gentili et al. 2011).

Most *RAPSYN* patients have little disability in the long run; the respiratory crises reduce in severity and frequency through the school years and are rarely seen in adulthood (Natera-de Benito et al. 2016) although there can still be some muscle fatigability later in childhood or early adulthood (Burke et al. 2003).

ChAT Mutations

ChAT mutations are classically known for causing neonatal-onset CMS with life-threatening or even fatal apnoeic episodes (Ohno et al. 2001). These episodes may require resuscitation at birth. Patients often have feeding difficulties due to deficits in sucking and swallowing – with the associated risk of aspiration. There is also a second phenotype with a later onset in infancy and childhood with apnoeic crises but a mild intercourse (Schara et al. 2010). The apnoeic crises can be precipitated by infections or stress or even excitement or overexertion (Ohno et al. 2001). There may be no obvious provoking trigger and there may be few or no other myasthenic symptoms (Engel et al. 2015); between crises they can have relatively normal muscle strength. The apnoeic episodes in *ChAT* mutations can require ventilatory support for many weeks. A few patients never breathe spontaneously and some develop hypoxaemic brain injury (Engel et al. 2015). Many patients improve slowly over time (even over the first few months of life) but severe episodes of apnoea and/or bulbar weakness can occur later in life.

Other Mutations

Many other mutations causing congenital myasthenia have been reported to cause childhood respiratory and bulbar complications (Table 9.3). Respiratory crises are rare in patients with AChR deficiency due to AChR ε-subunit mutations. Knowing the genotype/phenotype correlations allows proactive, anticipatory respiratory care, especially on the occurrence of an event that is known to trigger a worsening of the clinical situation. This is most important in the so called CMS-episodic apnoea (CMS-EA) forms, where severe life-threatening apnoeas can occur. This label is most commonly given to those forms caused by ChAT mutations but occur less commonly with *RAPSYN*, *SCN4A* (Mallory et al. 2009), *MYO9A*, *SLC5A7* and *SLC18A3* mutations (Lee et al. 2018).

Investigations

As with autoimmune myasthenia, all patients with congenital myasthenia, particularly those at risk of a crisis (e.g. younger ages and those with known triggers such as respiratory infections), should have regular assessments of respiratory function which should include observation of important clinical signs (Table 9.2). Otherwise the two most important respiratory investigations are spirometry and nocturnal sleep studies. Spirometry may show a reduced vital capacity and a restrictive defect due to respiratory

Table 9.3   Congenital myasthenic syndromes and their respiratory manifestations

Mutation	Reported respiratory/bulbar issues	Reference
COL13A1	Neonatal respiratory distress and feeding problems; pectus carinatum	Beeson et al. (2018)
COLQ	Early onset severe weakness and respiratory crises. Chronic hypoventilation with progressive respiratory muscle weakness needing long-term ventilatory support	Finlayson et al. (2013b); Robb et al. (2010)
DPAGT1	Occasional mild bulbar weakness; shortness of breath and reduced FVC (<70% predicted)	Finlayson et al. (2013a)
MYO9A	Severe neonatal presentation with respiratory and bulbar involvement	O'Connor et al. (2016)
LAMA5	Respiratory distress requiring tracheostomy	Maselli et al. (2018)
LAMB2	Severe neonatal respiratory distress	Maselli et al. (2009)
LRP4	Respiratory failure and feeding problems from shortly after birth	Ohkawara et al. (2014); Rodríguez Cruz et al. (2014)
MuSK	Neonatal respiratory failure requiring ventilation	Maselli et al. (2010)
PREPL	Weakness and feeding problems from birth	Régal et al. (2014)
SCN4A	3–30 minute bouts of neonatal respiratory distress and life threatening apnoeic episodes	Tsujino et al. (2003)
SLC5A7	Neonatal episodic apnoea	Lee et al. (2018)
SLC18A3	Episodic apnoeas	Lee et al. (2018)
Slow-channel CMS	Progressive respiratory muscle weakness and respiratory failure	Robb et al. (2010)

FVC, vital capacity.

muscle weakness; it may also be reduced during acute episodes (such as with infections) and can be used regularly during hospital admissions to monitor respiratory muscle strength.

Nocturnal sleep studies are essential as weakness of the upper airway and respiratory muscles in patients with CMS puts them at risk of sleep disordered breathing and nocturnal hypoventilation, especially during REM sleep. Sleep studies may however be normal between episodes in those patients that have sporadic, acute crises. Children with CMS can have markedly raised apnoea-hypopnoea and oxygen desaturation indices (Caggiano et al. 2017; Griffon et al. 2017). Hypoxaemia and hypercarbia would not be seen until ventilation fell below a certain threshold and ventilation will also often be normal while awake.

Treatments

All patients with congenital myasthenic syndromes should have a detailed respiratory care plan. Part of this plan should be open/fast-track access to their local tertiary paediatric centre. Early medical review should be sought in the event of respiratory infections with early recourse to antibiotics (and the use of antibiotics at home by parents if needed).

All children with CMS should be under the care of a respiratory paediatrician and have regular reviews including sleep studies as needed. Apnoea alarms may be useful in those at risk. If sleep studies show significant nocturnal hypoventilation then home NIV may be needed in the form of BiPAP. This may also be needed if children have certain mutations (e.g. COLQ due to its association with progressive respiratory muscle weakness) or have multiple episodes of respiratory failure (Robb et al. 2010). NIV can also be used during acute exacerbations before transfer to hospital. Some patients may also require support in the day to allow periods of rest. Inspiratory pressures of at least 14–18cm H_2O may be needed, together with a positive end expiratory pressure (PEEP) of 4cm and an age appropriate rate (Robb et al. 2010). The use of NIV for pre-crisis management has been very successful in some centres (Robb et al. 2010). The use of NIV should be regularly reviewed to ensure settings are correct and the interface device (e.g. face mask) is appropriate for the age and size of the child.

Invasive ventilation on a paediatric intensive care unit can be needed during particularly severe episodes. Tracheostomy may be required, either to facilitate long-term ventilation in those with severe hypoventilation (and to avoid the complications of long-term nasal/face masks) or due to bilateral vocal cord palsy. Ear Nose and Throat specialist review may be needed as tonsillar hypertrophy causing obstructive sleep apnoea can be associated with a respiratory crisis. Moderate tonsillar hypertrophy that would be less significant in children without neuromuscular disease can be much more clinically important in the face of respiratory muscle weakness.

Chest physiotherapy is essential, especially during infective episodes or acute crises. This may include the use of cough assist devices or lung volume recruitment bags to aid in airway secretion expectoration/removal.

Bulbar weakness and feeding/swallowing problems should be adequately treated due to the risk of aspiration. Expert swallowing assessments should be carried out by paediatric speech therapists and appropriate alterations made to feeding plans to minimise the risk of lung disease caused by aspiration. Glycopyrrolate or hyoscine can be used to treat excessive oropharyngeal secretions. Nutrition may need to be supported (in the short or long term) by nasogastric tube or gastrostomy feeding. Gastro-oesophageal reflux should also be aggressively managed.

Parents and carers should be taught resuscitation skills before patient discharge and these skills should be regularly refreshed. This teaching should involve the use of bag-valve-masks for those at risk of sudden acute deterioration. Parents should also be aware of the symptoms and signs indicating imminent respiratory crises; this is especially important in those with high risk genotypes (for example, those causing CMS-EA) and in those with a prior history of respiratory problems.

Patients should be fully immunised according to the relevant national schedule. This should include pneumococcal vaccination and the seasonal influenza vaccine.

REFERENCES

al Ahdal O, Bevan D (1995) Clindamycin-induced neuromuscular blockade. *Can J Anaesth* **42**: 614–617.

Amino A, Shiozawa Z, Nagasaka T et al. (1998) Sleep apnoea in well-controlled myasthenia gravis and the effect of thymectomy. *J Neurol* **245**: 77–80.

Anderson JA, Ng JJ, Bowe C et al. (2008) Variable phenotypes associated with mutations in DOK7. *Muscle Nerve* **37**: 448–456.

Andrews PI (2004) Autoimmune myasthenia gravis in childhood. *Semin Neurol* **24**: 101–110.

Argov Z, Brenner T, Abramsky O et al. 1986) Ampicillin may aggravate clinical and experimental myasthenia gravis. *Arch Neurol* **43**: 255–256.

Barrons RW (1997) Drug-induced neuromuscular blockade and myasthenia gravis. *Pharmacotherapy* **17**: 1220–1232.

Beeson D, Cossins J, Rodríguez Cruz P, Maxwell S, Liu WW, Palace J (2018) Myasthenic syndromes due to defects in COL13A1 and in the N-linked glycosylation pathway. *Ann N Y Acad Sci* **1413**: 163–169.

Ben Ammar A, Petit F, Alexandri N et al. (2010) Phenotype genotype analysis in 15 patients presenting a congenital myasthenic syndrome due to mutations in DOK7. *J Neurol* **257**: 754–766.

Beri S, Hussain N, Balky A, Alzoubidi R, Gosalakkal J, Kanhere S (2009) Bulbar dysfunction: an early presentation of congenital myasthenic syndrome. *Eur J Paediatr Neurol* **13(Suppl-1):** S46.

Bourke SC, Gibson GJ (2002) Sleep and breathing in neuromuscular disease. *Eur Respir J* **19:** 1194–1201.

Burke G, Cossins J, Maxwell S et al. (2003) Rapsyn mutations in hereditary myasthenia: distinct early- and late-onset phenotypes. *Neurology* **61:** 826–828.

Caggiano S, Khirani S, Verrillo E et al. (2017) Sleep in infants with congenital myasthenic syndromes. *Eur J Paed Neurol* **21:** 842–851.

Chiang LM, Darras BT, Kang PB (2009) Juvenile myasthenia gravis. *Muscle Nerve* **39:** 423–431.

Dushay KM, Zibrak JD, Jensen WA (1990) Myasthenia gravis presenting as isolated respiratory failure. *Chest* **97:** 232–234.

Elias SB, Butler I, Appel SH (1979) Neonatal myasthenia gravis in the infant of a myasthenic mother in remission. *Ann Neurol* **6:** 72–75.

Engel AG, Shen XM, Selcen D, Sine SM (2015) Congenital myasthenic syndromes: pathogenesis, diagnosis, and treatment. *Lancet Neurol* **14:** 420–434.

Evoli A, Tonali PA, Padua L et al. (2003) Clinical correlates with anti-MuSK antibodies in generalized seronegative myasthenia gravis. *Brain* **126:** 2304–2311.

Eymard B, Hantai D, Estournet B (2013) Congenital myasthenic syndromes. In: Dulac M, Lassonde M, Sarnat S (Eds), *Pediatric Neurology, Part III.* Handbook of Clinical Neurology 3rd edn., Volume 113. Burlington: Elsevier Science.

Finlayson S, Beeson D, Palace J (2013a) Congenital myasthenic syndromes: an update. *Pract Neurol* **13:** 80–91.

Finlayson S, Palace J, Belaya K et al. (2013b) Clinical features of congenital myasthenic syndrome due to mutations in DPAGT1. *J Neurol Neurosurg Psychiatry* **84:** 1119–1125.

Gadient P, Bolton J, Puri V (2009) Juvenile myasthenia gravis: three case reports and a literature review. *J Child Neurol* **24:** 584–590.

Gentili A, Ansaloni S, Morello W, Cecini MT, Cordelli DM, Baroncini S (2011) Diagnosis of congenital myasthenic syndrome with mutation of the RAPSN gene after general anaesthesia. *Eur J Anaesthesiol* **28:** 748–749.

Griffon L, Amaddeo A, Mortamet G et al. (2017) Sleep study as a diagnostic tool for unexplained respiratory failure in infants hospitalized in the PICU. *J Crit Care* **42:** 317–323.

Griggs RC, Donohoe KM, Utell MJ, Goldblatt D, Moxley RT III (1981) Evaluation of pulmonary function in neuromuscular disease. *Arch Neurol* **38:** 9–12.

Hutchison AA, Russell G (1979) Respiratory studies in an infant with neonatal myasthenia gravis. *Aust Paediatr J* **15:** 44–46.

Jennett AM, Bali D, Jasti P, Shah B, Browning LA (2006) Telithromycin and myasthenic crisis. *Clin Infect Dis* **43:** 1621–1622.

Jephson CG, Mills NA, Pitt MC et al. (2010) Congenital stridor with feeding difficulty as a presenting symptom of Dok7 congenital myasthenic syndrome. *Int J Pediatr Otorhinolaryngol* **74:** 991–994.

Jones SC, Sorbello A, Boucher RM (2011) Fluoroquinolone-associated myasthenia gravis exacerbation: evaluation of postmarketing reports from the United States FDA adverse event reporting system and a literature review. *Drug Saf* **34:** 839–847.

Jovandaric MZ, Despotovic DJ, Jesic MM, Jesic MD (2016) Neonatal outcome in pregnancies with autoimmune myasthenia gravis. *Fetal Pediatr Pathol* **35:** 167–172.

Kataoka H, Kiriyama T, Kawaguchi T et al. (2014) Preoperative low-dose steroid can prevent respiratory insufficiency after thymectomy in generalized myasthenia gravis. *Eur Neurol* **72:** 228–233.

Keenan SP, Alexander D, Road JD, Ryan CF, Oger J, Wilcox PG (1995) Ventilatory muscle strength and endurance in myasthenia gravis. *Eur Respir J* **8:** 1130–1135.

Kinali M, Beeson D, Pitt MC et al. (2008) Congenital myasthenic syndromes in childhood: diagnostic and management challenges. *J Neuroimmunol* **201–202:** 6–12.

Lai YC, Chen JY, Wu HD, Yang CC, Lin CH, Lee PL (2016) Sleep disordered breathing mimicking myasthenia grisis in a patient with myasthenia gravis. *J Clin Sleep Med* **12:** 767–769.

Lee M, Beeson D, Palace J (2018) Therapeutic strategies for congenital myasthenic syndromes. *Ann N Y Acad Sci* **1412:** 129–136.

Lindstrom JM, Lennon VA, Seybold ME, Whittingham S (1976) Experimental autoimmune myasthenia gravis and myasthenia gravis: biochemical and immunochemical aspects. *Ann N Y Acad Sci* **274:** 254–274.

Mallory LA, Shaw JG, Burgess SL et al. (2009) Congenital myasthenic syndrome with episodic apnea. *Pediatr Neurol* **41:** 42–45.

Manni R, Piccolo G, Sartori I et al. (1995) Breathing during sleep in myasthenia gravis. *Ital J Neurol Sci* **16:** 589–594.

Maselli RA, Ng JJ, Anderson JA et al. (2009) Mutations in LAMB2 causing a severe form of synaptic congenital myasthenic syndrome. *J Med Genet* **46:** 203–208.

Maselli RA, Arredondo J, Cagney O et al. (2010) Mutations in MUSK causing congenital myasthenic syndrome impair MuSK-Dok-7 interaction. *Hum Mol Genet* **19:** 2370–2379.

Maselli RA, Arredondo J, Vázquez J et al. (2018) A presynaptic congenital myasthenic syndrome attributed to a homozygous sequence variant in LAMA5. *Ann N Y Acad Sci* **1413:** 119–125.

McQuillen MP, Cantor HE, O'Rourke JR (1968) Myasthenic syndrome associated with antibiotics. *Arch Neurol* **18:** 402–415.

Müller JS, Herczegfalvi A, Vilchez JJ et al. (2007) Phenotypical spectrum of DOK7 mutations in congenital myasthenic syndromes. *Brain* **130:** 1497–1506.

Natera-de Benito D, Bestué M, Vilchez JJ et al. (2016) Long-term follow-up in patients with congenital myasthenic syndrome due to RAPSN mutations. *Neuromuscul Disord* **26:** 153–159.

O'Connor E, Töpf A, Müller JS et al. (2016) Identification of mutations in the MYO9A gene in patients with congenital myasthenic syndrome. *Brain* **139:** 2143–2153.

Ohkawara B, Cabrera-Serrano M, Nakata T et al. (2014) LRP4 third β-propeller domain mutations cause novel congenital myasthenia by compromising agrin-mediated MuSK signalling in a position-specific manner. *Hum Mol Genet* **23:** 1856–1868.

Ohno K, Tsujino A, Brengman JM et al. (2001) Choline acetyltransferase mutations cause myasthenic syndrome associated with episodic apnea in humans. *Proc Natl Acad Sci USA* **98:** 2017–2022.

O'Riordan J, Javed M, Doherty C, Hutchinson M (1994) Worsening of myasthenia gravis on treatment with imipenem/cilastatin. *J Neurol Neurosurg Psychiatry* **57:** 383.

Palace J, Lashley D, Bailey S et al. (2012) Clinical features in a series of fast channel congenital myasthenia syndrome. *Neuromuscul Disord* **22:** 112–117.

Papazian O (1992) Transient neonatal myasthenia gravis. *J Child Neurol* **7:** 135–141.

Peragallo JH (2017) Pediatric myasthenia gravis. *Semin Pediatr Neurol* **24:** 116–121.

Pfeffer G, Povitz M, Gibson GJ, Chinnery PF (2015) Diagnosis of muscle diseases presenting with early respiratory failure. *J Neurol* **262:** 1101–1114.

Piastra M, Conti G, Caresta E et al. (2005) Noninvasive ventilation options in pediatric myasthenia gravis. *Paediatr Anaesth* **15:** 699–702.

Popperud TH, Boldingh MI, Rasmussen M, Kerty E (2017) Juvenile myasthenia gravis in Norway: clinical characteristics, treatment, and long-term outcome in a nationwide population-based cohort. *Eur J Paediatr Neurol* **21:** 707–714.

Quera-Salva MA, Guilleminault C, Chevret S et al. (1992) Breathing disorders during sleep in myasthenia gravis. *Ann Neurol* **31:** 86–92.

Qureshi AI, Choundry MA, Mohammad Y, Chua HC, Yahia AM, Ulatowski JA et al. (2004) Respiratory failure as a first presentation of myasthenia gravis. *Med Sci Monit* **10:** CR684–CR689.

Rabinstein AA (2005) Update on respiratory management of critically ill neurologic patients. *Curr Neurol Neurosci Rep* **5:** 476–482.

Rabinstein A, Wijdicks EF (2002) BiPAP in acute respiratory failure due to myasthenic crisis may prevent intubation. *Neurology* **59:** 1647–1649.

Rabinstein AA, Mueller-Kronast N (2005) Risk of extubation failure in patients with myasthenic crisis. *Neurocrit Care* **3:** 213–215.

Régal L, Shen XM, Selcen D et al. (2014) PREPL deficiency with or without cystinuria causes a novel myasthenic syndrome. *Neurology* **82:** 1254–1260.

Richman DP, Agius MA (2003) Treatment of autoimmune myasthenia gravis. *Neurology* **61:** 1652–1661.

Rieder P, Louis M, Jolliet P, Chevrolet JC (1995) The repeated measurement of vital capacity is a poor predictor of the need for mechanical ventilation in myasthenia gravis. *Intensive Care Med* **21:** 663–668.

Robb SA, Muntoni F, Simonds AK (2010) Respiratory Management of Congenital Myasthenic Syndromes in Childhood: Workshop, 8th December 2009; UCL Institute of Neurology, London, UK. *Neuromuscul Disord* **20:** 833–838.

Rodríguez Cruz PM, Palace J, Beeson D (2014) Congenital myasthenic syndromes and the neuromuscular junction. *Curr Opin Neurol* **27:** 566–575.

Sanders DB, El-Salem K, Massey JM, McConville J, Vincent A (2003) Clinical aspects of MuSK antibody positive seronegative MG. *Neurology* **60:** 1978–1980.

Sanders DB, Wolfe GI, Benatar M et al. (2016) International consensus guidance for management of myasthenia gravis: executive summary. *Neurology* **87:** 419–425.

Schakman O, Gilson H, Thissen JP (2008) Mechanisms of glucocorticoid-induced myopathy. *J Endocrinol* **197:** 1–10.

Schara U, Christen HJ, Durmus H et al. (2010) Long-term follow-up in patients with congenital myasthenic syndrome due to ChAT mutations. *Eur J Paediatr Neurol* **14:** 326–333.

Seneviratne J, Mandrekar J, Wijdicks EF, Rabinstein AA (2008a) Noninvasive ventilation in myasthenic crisis. *Arch Neurol* **65:** 54–58.

Seneviratne J, Mandrekar J, Wijdicks EF, Rabinstein AA (2008b) Predictors of extubation failure in myasthenic crisis. *Arch Neurol* **65:** 929–933.

Seok HY, Shin HY, Kim JK et al. (2017) The impacts of influenza infection and vaccination on exacerbation of myasthenia gravis. *J Clin Neurol* **13:** 325–330.

Tackenberg B, Schneider M, Blaes F et al. (2018) Acetylcholine receptor antibody titers and clinical course after influenza vaccination in patients with myasthenia gravis: a double-blind randomized controlled trial (ProPATIent-Trial). *EBioMedicine* **28:** 143–150.

Thomas CE, Mayer SA, Gungor Y et al. (1997) Myasthenic crisis: clinical features, mortality, complications, and risk factors for prolonged intubation. *Neurology* **48:** 1253–1260.

Tsujino A, Maertens C, Ohno K et al. (2003) Myasthenic syndrome caused by mutation of the SCN4A sodium channel. *Proc Natl Acad Sci USA* **100:** 7377–7382.

Unal O, Teber S, Kendirli T, Deda G, Anlar B (2007) Juvenile form of myasthenia gravis presenting as recurrent pulmonary infection with atelectasis. *Pediatr Int* **49:** 1007–1008.

Vachharajani A, Uong EC (2005) The role of polysomnography in the diagnosis of a neuromuscular disorder. *J Clin Sleep Med* **1:** 398–399.

Varelas PN, Chua HC, Natterman J et al. (2002) Ventilatory care in myasthenia gravis crisis: assessing the baseline adverse event rate. *Crit Care Med* **30:** 2663–2668.

Verspyck E, Mandelbrot L, Dommergues M et al. (1993) Myasthenia gravis with polyhydramnios in the fetus of an asymptomatic mother. *Prenat Diagn* **13:** 539–542.

Watanabe A, Watanabe T, Obama T et al. (2004) Prognostic factors for myasthenic crisis after transsternal thymectomy in patients with myasthenia gravis. *J Thorac Cardiovasc Surg* **127:** 868–876.

Wittbrodt ET (1997) Drugs and myasthenia gravis. An update. *Arch Intern Med* **157:** 399–408.

Therapy and Exercise in Myasthenia

Hayley Ramjattan

INTRODUCTION

Congenital myasthenic syndromes (CMS) are a group of rare genetic disorders affecting the neuromuscular junction (NMJ) structure and function (Finlayson et al. 2013). They are characterised by the presence of fatigable muscle weakness, but age at onset, presenting symptoms, distribution of weakness, and response to treatment differ depending on the molecular mechanism that results from the genetic defect (Rodríguez Cruz et al. 2014). The severity of CMS is highly variable amongst individuals and can fluctuate and worsen with physical effort, which makes assessing for and prescribing graded exercise a challenge for this population. (Angelini 2014).

Myasthenia gravis is an autoimmune disease affecting the NMJ, and is characterised by painless fatigable muscle weakness, as a result of antibodies targeted at the NMJ proteins (Jacob et al. 2009). Myasthenia gravis exhibits the same physiological mechanism of fatigability as CMS, but exercise advice is often given with even greater caution, due to the high risk of worsening physical symptoms with over-activity before it is well controlled.

There is limited research on the effects of exercise participation in the CMS population which may in part be due to the rarity of the condition and its heterogeneity. The effects of exercise on patients with myasthenia gravis has interested medical professionals for some time with laboratory assays of cholinesterase levels after muscular exercise (Stoner and Wilson 1943). However, there is some published evidence on the benefits of exercise programmes and physiotherapy for adults with myasthenia gravis (Cass 2013). These are mainly limited to single case reports (Stout et al. 2001; Davidson et al. 2005; Lucia et al. 2007; Scheer et al. 2012); however, there a few studies, that successfully utilised graded exercise programmes in adults with myasthenia gravis (Lohi et al. 1993; Rahbek et al. 2017) which could be suitable for the older child with myasthenia.

EXERCISE IN MYASTHENIA – IS IT BENEFICIAL OR HARMFUL?

Exercise has many benefits in children, including developing self-confidence, limiting weight gain and offering a platform to learn new skills. It can also form part of a healthy lifestyle, promoting good habits which will carry over in to adulthood. However, strenuous aerobic exercise is often avoided in individuals with myasthenia due to the negative consequences of muscle fatigability. Rest is recommended during acute exacerbations or in the face of frequent fatigue whilst engaging in activities of daily life. There is lack of an evidence base for the benefits of exercise during interim fatigue-free periods during the natural course of the disease.

There is even less research on the effects of exercise in children with myasthenia, although adult studies evidence improvements in maximal muscle strength, patient confidence and greater functional capacity, following a progressive resistance training programme, with no worsening of myasthenic symptoms (Rahbek et al. 2017; Westerberg et al. 2017). There is also evidence to support better surgical outcomes and reduce hospital admission in patients undergoing thymectomy who receive pre-operative and post-operative physical rehabilitation (Ambrogi and Mineo 2017). Systematic reviews of exercise therapy in a host of neuromuscular disorders have previously shown Level 3 evidence for effectiveness of aerobic exercise in muscle disorders and for breathing exercises for patients with myasthenia gravis in adults (Cup et al. 2007).

Children with myasthenia gravis are often managed with steroids, which can predispose them to significant weight gain. A systematic review by García-Hermoso et al. (2018) concluded that a combination of aerobic and resistance training offers greater health benefits to obese children than aerobic training alone. Rahbek et al. (2017) also demonstrated that aerobic training, plus progressive resistance training was superior to aerobic activity alone in adults with myasthenia gravis, resulting in increase in muscle strength and functional capacity. These findings could be applied to guiding activity programmes for the myasthenic child experiencing weight gain.

In children with myasthenia gravis, early guidance following acute onset of crisis is important to support their return to normal function as soon as possible. When prescribing exercise, it is important to be cautious; pacing of activities is key and should be planned in tandem with medication management. Muscle cramps and exercise-induced myalgia are often reported in individuals with myasthenia. These can be successfully managed with massage and stretching advice, and careful application of heat.

WHAT EXERCISE IS RECOMMENDED IN MYASTHENIA?

Children with myasthenia should not avoid exercise and instead an age-appropriate exercise program and activity advice should be given and monitored closely. Knowledge of normal motor development is essential in supporting acquisition of motor skills in the younger developing child and clear goals should be identified in collaboration with the child and parents.

The type of activity or exercise advised will depend on the child's age and type of myasthenia. Young children with RAPSYN CMS often experience respiratory crisis in early infancy, decreasing in frequency and severity with age (Natera-de Benito et al. 2016). Therefore, activity to promote motor skill development may be delayed until they are medically stable. For other infants, the early stages of motor development may be delayed due to muscle weakness and the repetition required to learn a new skill may be limited by fatigue. These children may require additional aids and physiotherapy to support their development.

Activity pacing is a key element of an established exercise programme and the child/family will be aware of the signs of fatigue such as ptosis, slurred speech and breathing changes. Activity plans should be adhered to and monitored and keeping an activity diary may be of benefit to identify any times of increased fatigue.

Lohi et al. (1993) and Davidson et al. (2005) both evaluated strength programmes in adults with mild to moderate myasthenia gravis and demonstrated the need for caution when prescribing the number of repetitions. Their subjects were frequently unable to complete the prescribed number of repetitions and would self-limit their activity. Children are often unable to limit their activity in the same way and caution should be given when advising on repeated activities. Management of the child's physical abilities must involve a combination of optimal medication and guidance on pacing physical activities.

PHYSIOTHERAPY IN MYASTHENIA

A detailed history is required before advising physical activity in children with myasthenia. This includes timing of medication and any recent changes to the individual's regime. A child's medication regime is often altered to reflect changes in function and can be adjusted at times of growth, puberty and illness. Certain medications work fast on reversing the effects of myasthenia and others take longer to establish in the system. In congenital myasthenia, medications may take several months to repair the damage to the motor endplate. Knowledge of the medications and time since last dose as well as the time needed for some medications to improve function optimally will be important when you assess a child and recommend a regime of exercise.

Mobility

The physiotherapist must consider the age-appropriate motor development of the child. A detailed history of early years' development will highlight risk of contractures or weakness, and identify any recent medical events that may have caused immobility.

The physiotherapist should ascertain the child's current functional baseline, including any recent fluctuations (e.g. within the last 4 weeks). Several factors can affect a child's function and mobility, including stress, temperature, hormonal changes, recent levels of activity, timing and changes to medication. An assessment may include details of their current level of ambulation, the distance the child is able to walk before fatigue, and changes to their gait pattern with prolonged walking. Wheelchair use should be noted, including when and how often it is required.

Children with myasthenia may fatigue quickly and it is important to keep the number of assessments performed to a minimum, ensuring they are standardised and relevant to the individual. Make sure they are fully supported in between each physical task you ask them to do. There are currently no widely available diseasespecific assessments appropriate to use in children with myasthenia. Adult scoring systems are often unreliable in children due to reduced cooperation and developmental limitations, and modified versions should be used to monitor treatment efficacy (Parr et al. 2010). Timed tests can be very useful in evaluating the effectiveness of therapy intervention and medication. Repeated tests help highlight any muscle fatigability and may include; timed rise from the floor, 10metre run/walk and the number of sit to stands performed in a minute. Jordan et al. (2017) demonstrated use of both repetitive limb movement and 6-minute walk test to be effective in identifying muscle fatigue in adults and could be used with the older child. Muscle myometry is a sensitive method of identifying changes in limb strength (Vinge and Andersen 2016) and should be used where available.

Fatigable muscle weakness can fluctuate throughout the day, affecting all muscle groups, including the respiratory muscles. Muscles of the face and mouth can fatigue causing droopy eyelids, slurred speech and difficulties chewing and swallowing. These features may be early warning signs of a child's over-activity. However, it is important to recognise the difference between general fatigue and muscle fatigue. Patient reported fatigue with the absence of muscle weakness should be treated with caution and may indicate the need for a bio-psychosocial approach.

Exercise-induced myalgia is occasionally reported in children with myasthenia, although pain is not a key feature and can be associated with increased patient activity levels, muscle imbalance or injury. Location, duration, intensity, aggravating and easing factors are all important to assess when patients report pain. The use of a pain diary may be of benefit.

Posture and Spine

Visualisation and palpation of the spine, noting trunk and neck position should be carried out in both sitting and standing. Not all children with myasthenia will develop a scoliosis, but children with CMS COLQ can frequently present with severe and progressive weakness from birth or early infancy (Rodríguez

Cruz et al. 2014), leading to postural asymmetry. Be mindful that children may develop idiopathic scoliosis, separate from their underlying muscle weakness. Early management of the spine is essential, including education on postural habits, both at home and in school, and good seating options especially in the very weak and fatigued child. A small number of children with myasthenia will require spinal surgery. Preoperative planning and post-operative management will need to be considered, ensuring adequate support is available for likely post-operative fatigue.

Limbs/joint Range of Movement

Contractures can develop due to reduced mobility and prolonged static postures. In the weaker infant who sits for prolonged periods of time, it is particularly important to note hip extension, knee extension and ankle dorsiflexion, as this can impact on a child's ability to walk. Any differences between passive and active range of movement should be noted, highlighting areas of muscle weakness. Management options may include targeted stretches, orthotics, postural management, activity and exercise. Balance strategy training multimodal exercise was shown to improve balance and functional mobility in adults with myasthenia gravis (Wong et al. 2014). Similar programmes designed for children appropriate to their level of physical developmental age may be of some benefit. Treatment with steroids in particular may predispose children to osteoporosis with easy fractures. They should be handled carefully. Long-term use of steroids can also affect growth in children and should be monitored carefully.

Respiratory and Bulbar Function

Children with all types of myasthenia can have difficulties with their breathing, speaking and bulbar function. Children with myasthenia gravis can occasionally present in myasthenic crisis, leading to impairment of their respiratory muscles, necessitating ventilatory support (Finnis and Jayawant 2011). Recognising the specific subtypes of CMS that are at higher risk can be important for early detection and guiding medical management. Respiratory function can be severely compromised in infants with RAPSYN CMS (Natera-de Benito et al. 2016) but often improves to near normal after the first 2 years of life. Assessment and provision of respiratory support can be a key adjunct in a child's therapy. Forced vital capacity (FVC) is often a good indicator of respiratory muscle weakness in the older child (Hull 2012).

Children with myasthenia may also be at risk of having chewing and swallowing difficulties leading to choking or aspiration. These can be ascertained by taking a detailed history from the patient or parent and timely referrals on to relevant services. Knowledge and application of secretion clearance techniques taught by the physiotherapist are important. Children with myasthenia are susceptible to quick deterioration in their respiratory function and timely intervention is key to effective management.

OCCUPATIONAL THERAPY INPUT TO IMPROVE ACTIVITIES OF DAILY LIVING AND QUALITY OF LIFE AT HOME AND SCHOOL

Occupational therapy can play a key role in educating adults supporting the child, about the effects of myasthenia and strategies to help manage fatigue. Timely referrals, can be key in supporting a child's access and independence, including environmental adaptations and wheelchair use.

Children with myasthenia often have visual difficulties due to restricted eye movements – diplopia (double vision) or ptosis (eye lid closure) – therefore; positioning in the classroom needs to be optimal. Neck weakness and muscle fatigue can be caused by continual looking down and up (e.g. from the whiteboard at school). An occupational therapist should help advise on ways to reduce this with the use of aids (e.g. interactive tablet, sloping board), seating and advice on optimal placement in the classroom environment.

Children should be provided with suitable mobility equipment to support optimal participation in life. This may include walking aids to support motor skill acquisition when young and a timely referral to wheelchair service. Assessment and provision of an appropriate wheelchair is important to support the child's independence, taking special note of head posture to accommodate possible altered vision and neck weakness. Regular assessment is required to ensure the child accommodates a symmetrical posture and adequate support, to help limit fatigue.

Advice and education provision to a child's nursery, school or college about myasthenia can be hugely beneficial in supporting a child's access to the curriculum. Appropriate inclusion of physical education and games activities will be essential in supporting the child's participation in school activities. If feeding concerns are present, patients will need speech and language therapy input and may need guidance on altered meals and longer lunch times at school.

REFERENCES

Ambrogi V, Mineo TC (2017) Benefits of comprehensive rehabilitation therapy in thymectomy for myasthenia gravis: a propensity score matching analysis. *Am J Phys Med Rehabil* **96**: 77–83.

Angelini C (2014) Congenital myasthenic syndrome. In: Angelini, C (Ed.), *Genetic Neuromuscular Disorders: A Case-Based Approach*. Springer International Publishing, pp. 195–197.

Birnbaum S, Hogrel JY, Porcher R et al. (2018) The benefits and tolerance of exercise in myasthenia gravis (MGEX): study protocol for a randomised controlled trial. *Trials* **19**: 49.

Cass S (2013) Myasthenia gravis and sports participation. *Curr Sports Med Rep* **12**: 18–21.

Cup EH, Pieterse AJ, Ten Broek-Pastoor JM et al. (2007) Exercise therapy and other types of physical therapy for patients with neuromuscular diseases: a systematic review. *Arch Phys Med Rehabil* **88**: 1452–1464.

Davidson L, Hale L, Mulligan H (2005) Exercise prescription in the physiotherapeutic management of myasthenia gravis: a case report. *N Z J Physiother* **33**: 13–18.

Finlayson S, Beeson D, Palace J (2013) Congenital myasthenic syndromes: an update. *Pract Neurol* **13**: 80–91. Finnis M, Jayawant S (2011) Juvenile myasthenia gravis: a paediatric perspective. *Autoimmune Dis* **2011**: 404101.

García-Hermoso A, Ramírez-Vélez R, RamírezCampillo R, Peterson M, Martínez-Vizcaíno V (2018) Concurrent aerobic plus resistance exercise versus aerobic exercise alone to improve health outcomes in paediatric obesity: a systematic review and meta-analysis. *Br J Sports Med* **52**: 161–166.

Hull J (2012) British Thoracic Society guideline for respiratory management of children with neuromuscular weakness: commentary. *Thorax* **67**: 654–655.

Jacob S, Viegas S, Lashley D, Hilton-Jones D (2009) Myasthenia gravis and other neuromuscular junction disorders. *Pract Neurol* **9**: 364–371.

Jordan B, Mehl T, Schweden TLK, Menge U, Zierz S (2017) Assessment of physical fatigability and fatigue perception in myasthenia gravis. *Muscle Nerve* **55**: 657–663.

Lucia A, Maté-Muñoz JL, Pérez M, Foster C, Gutiérrez-Rivas E, Arenas J (2007) Double trouble (McArdle's disease and myasthenia gravis): How can exercise help? *Muscle Nerve* **35**: 125–128.

Lohi EL, Lindberg C, Andersen O (1993) Physical training effects in myasthenia gravis. *Arch Phys Med Rehabil* **74**: 1178–1180.

Natera-de Benito D, Bestué M, Vilchez JJ et al. (2016) Long-term follow-up in patients with congenital myasthenic syndrome due to RAPSN mutations. *Neuromuscul Disord* **26**: 153–159.

Parr J, Jayawant S, Buckley C, Vincent A (2010) *Childhood Autoimmune Myasthenia. Inflammatory and Autoimmune Disorders of the Nervous System in Children*. London: Mac Keith Press.

Rahbek MA, Mikkelsen EE, Overgaard K, Vinge L, Andersen H, Dalgas U (2017) Exercise in myasthenia gravis: A feasibility study of aerobic and resistance training. *Muscle Nerve* **56:** 700–709.

Rodríguez Cruz PM, Palace J, Beeson D (2014) Inherited disorders of the neuromuscular junction: an update. *J Neurol* **261(11):** 2234–2243.

Scheer BV, Valero-Burgos E, Costa R (2012) Myasthenia gravis and endurance exercise. *Am J Phys Med Rehabil* **91:** 725–727.

Stoner HB, Wilson A (1943) The effect of muscular exercise on the serum cholinesterase level in normal adults and in patients with myasthenia gravis. *J Physiol* **102:** 1–4.

Stout JR, Eckerson JM, May E, Coulter C, Bradley-Popovich GE (2001) Effects of resistance exercise and creatine supplementation on myasthenia gravis: a case study. *Med Sci Sports Exerc* **33:** 869–872.

Westerberg E, Molin CJ, Lindblad I, Emtner M, Punga AR (2017) Physical exercise in myasthenia gravis is safe and improves neuromuscular parameters and physical performance-based measures: A pilot study. *Muscle Nerve* **56:** 207–214.

Wong SH, Nitz JC, Williams K, Brauer SG (2014) Effects of balance strategy training in myasthenia gravis: a case study series. *Muscle Nerve* **49:** 654–660.

Vinge L, Andersen H (2016) Muscle strength and fatigue in newly diagnosed patients with myasthenia gravis. *Muscle Nerve* **54:** 709–714.

Transition of Care in Myasthenia

Sithara Ramdas and David Hilton-Jones

Transition in healthcare is defined as "the purposeful, planned movement of adolescents and young adults with chronic physical and medical conditions from child centred to adult-oriented health care systems" (Blum et al. 1993). It is well recognised that mortality and morbidity from chronic illness is increased when individuals move from paediatric to adult services (Tomlinson and Sugarman 1995; Somerville 1997; Watson 2000; Kipps et al. 2002; Bryden et al. 2003).

Transition of health care into adult services has long been thought of as a one-stop event. However this is now routinely recognised as a "transfer of care". Transition in fact is a journey through many stages and transfer of care is just one stage of this journey. This journey should be effective in gradually equipping the young person with the skills necessary to manage their own health care in both paediatric and adult services (Blum et al. 1993).

CHALLENGES TO TRANSITION

There are several challenges that must be recognised in ensuring a smooth and efficient transition. First and foremost is the anxiety associated with the loss of longstanding relationships that the young person and their family have had with health professionals. In a paediatric setting the health focus of a child/young person is viewed in context of the family. The shift of practice to an adult "individual" oriented setting can be challenging for the young person and their families. Family members might perceive themselves as having a diminished role in their child's health needs and will required support and guidance through this journey. Time constraints, language and cultural differences can all be barriers to ensuring a smooth transition.

The young person's knowledge of their condition, its progression and management are important to establish early in the journey, so that timely support can be offered.

APPROACHING TRANSITION

A planned co-ordinated approach, with the young person at the centre, is crucial to any transition process (Blum 1991; Bronheim et al. 1993). An adult physician or team that is both interested and capable of providing care is essential (Bronheim et al. 1993). Discussion between the paediatric and adult team, including a detailed summary of the young person's medical and social history, will empower the adult team to support the young person's transition of care and create an ethos of trust. Transition will take a variety of forms in different settings and could be led by one professional or the young person. It is important that all members of the team recognise their role in supporting transition to ensure a cohesive approach.

The actual timing of transfer of care can vary and needs to be individualised for a young person. Cognitive maturity of the young person, stability of the disease or any crucial impending changes in life can influence when this happens (Court 1991). In the years leading up to transfer of care, a young person should be encouraged to take on greater responsibility of their health, with the family concomitantly slowly shifting their role to advocates with less direct responsibility (Rosen 1993). Transition should be a holistic programme that addresses not only the young person's medical needs but additional issues like education, employment, relationships, independent living and social supports (Shaw et al. 2014). Effective transition has been shown to improve long-term outcome (Duguépéroux et al. 2008; Harden et al. 2012; Prestidge et al. 2012). The young person should be empowered and supported to have a clear voice during this process. They have the right to be involved in discussions and make informed decisions about their care (NICE 2016).

As much as for the young person, transition can be a challenging time for parents and carers as well. A systematic review on the outcomes and experiences of transition found that parents had higher levels of concern than young people (Coyne et al. 2017). Parents report their perceived concerns about their child's self-caring abilities related to the disease, and find it difficult to adapt into a new role with less involvement in their child's care (Craig et al. 2007; Iles and Lowton 2010). Discussion with families well ahead of time and providing them with sufficient information about the transition process is important to help families though this period of reported "turmoil".

Congenital myasthenia and juvenile myasthenia gravis (JMG) are lifelong conditions, though a proportion of children with both these conditions can go into remission and not require treatment in adult life. Young people with myasthenia are cognitively normal and so it is crucial they are well supported to be fully functioning productive members of society.

Some important issues which may need to addressed around transition are outlined in the following sections.

Motor Function

In children with congenital myasthenic syndrome (CMS), during pubertal growth spurts, it is common to see an apparent deterioration in muscle strength. In most cases once growth spurt is completed, the functional abilities return to previous levels.

Education

It is well recognised that the level of education is a significant predictor in long-term employment opportunities (van Mechelen et al. 2008; Minis et al. 2009, 2010). This is in particular in those with physical disabilities with normal cognition as they are likely to be in a more competitive employment market. Transition time is also the time around which the young person may be making the first move away from home to college or university. They are unlikely to have the same level of support and supervision of their families as they had during school years. Hence, it is important they feel empowered to able to express their wishes and highlight their physical difficulties, so that adaptations where necessary can be made to their day to day environment. It is important to ensure that they are not at any disadvantage compared to their physically able peers.

Medication

Certain types of CMS, such as RAPSYN CMS, improve throughout childhood and some adolescence and young adults may be able to reduce medication.

Compliance with Treatment

Compliance can be an issue especially in teenage years. In cases of unexplained deterioration compliance issues need to be suspected and addressed. Experiencing side-effects of steroids in particular may give rise to compliance issues.

Puberty

CMS and medication used to treat it do not affect puberty. JMG per se does not affect puberty but long-term steroid use can delay puberty, so teenagers on long-term steroids should be monitored to ensure that puberty is progressing as expected for age.

Sexual Health

Oral contraceptives can be used in CMS and autoimmune myasthenia. Pyridostigmine, salbutamol, 3,4-DAP, prednisolone and azathioprine are generally regarded to be safe in pregnancy.

Genetic Counselling

Except for slow-channel CMS which is autosomal dominant, all other types of CMS are autosomal recessive. However, in some populations where there is high level of consanguinity there is a higher possibility of having an affected child. Children who are becoming young adults need to be counselled regarding risks of inheritance depending on their sub-type of congenital myasthenia. This empowers them as young adults to make informed choices and decisions.

A transition checklist document, such as the Ready, Steady, Go programme, can be a helpful tool in the journey for the adolescent, their family and supporting health professionals (Nagra et al. 2015). It can be used as a guide to assess the young person's understanding of their condition and its implications on their day to day life. It also provides the young person the opportunity to ask specific questions which they may not do in a routine clinic appointment. This checklist can be a useful document for the adult team to identify areas of need and on-going support for the young person.

REFERENCES

Blum RW (1991) Overview of transition issues for youth with disabilities. *Pediatrician* **18:** 101–104.

Bronheim S, Fie S, Schidlow D, Magrab P, Boczar K, Dillon C (1993) *Crossings: A Manual for Transition of Chronically Ill Youth to Adult Health Care.* Pennsylvania: Bureau of Maternal and Child Health, Pennsylvania Department of Health.

Blum RW, Garell D, Hodgman CH et al. (1993) Transition from child-centered to adult health-care systems for adolescents with chronic conditions. A position paper of the Society for Adoles- cent Medicine. *J Adolesc Health* **14:** 570–576.

Bryden KS, Dunger DB, Mayou RA, Peveler RC, Neil HA (2003) Poor prognosis of young adults with type 1 diabetes: a longitudinal study. *Diabetes Care* **26:** 1052–1057.

Court JM (1991) Outpatient-based transition services for youth. *Pediatrician* **18:** 150–156.

Coyne I, Sheehan AM, Heery E, While AE (2017) Improving transition to adult healthcare for young people with cystic fibrosis: A systematic review. *J Child Health Care* **21:** 312–330.

Craig SL, Towns S, Bibby H (2007) Moving on from paediatric to adult health care: an initial evaluation of a transition program for young people with cystic fibrosis. *Int J Adolesc Med Health* **19:** 333–343.

Duguépéroux I, Tamalet A, Sermet-Gaudelus I et al. (2008) Clinical changes of patients with cystic fibrosis during transition from pediatric to adult care. *J Adolesc Health* **43**: 459–465.

Harden PN, Walsh G, Bandler N et al. (2012) Bridging the gap: an integrated paediatric to adult clinical service for young adults with kidney failure. *BMJ* **344**: e3718.

Iles N, Lowton K (2010) What is the perceived nature of parental care and support for young people with cystic fibrosis as they enter adult health services? *Health Soc Care Community* **18**: 21–29.

Kipps S, Bahu T, Ong K et al. (2002) Current methods of transfer of young people with Type 1 diabetes to adult services. *Diabet Med* **19**: 649–654.

Minis M-AH, Kalkman JS, Akkermans RP et al. (2010) Employment status of patients with neuromuscular diseases in relation to personal factors, fatigue and health status: a secondary analysis. *J Rehabil Med* **42**: 60–65.

Minis MA, Heerkens Y, Engels J, Oostendorp R, van Engelen B (2009) Classification of employment factors according to the International Classification of Functioning, Disability and Health in patients with neuromuscular diseases: a systematic review. *Disabil Rehabil* **31**: 2150–2163.

Nagra A, McGinnity PM, Davis N, Salmon AP (2015) Implementing transition: Ready Steady Go. *Arch Dis Child Educ Pract Ed* **100**: 313–320.

NICE (2016) Transition from children's to adults' services for young people using health or social care services. NICE guideline [NG43]. London: NICE. Available at: www.nice.org.uk/guidance/ng43.

Prestidge C, Romann A, Djurdjev O, Matsuda-Abedini M (2012) Utility and cost of a renal transplant transition clinic. *Pediatr Nephrol* **27**: 295–302.

Rosen DS (1993) Transition to adult health care for adolescents and young adults with cancer. *Cancer* **71(Suppl)**: 3411–3414.

Shaw KL, Watanabe A, Rankin E, McDonagh JE (2014) Walking the talk. Implementation of transitional care guidance in a UK paediatric and a neighbouring adult facility. *Child Care Health Dev* **40**: 663–670.

Somerville J (1997) Management of adults with congenital heart disease: an increasing problem. *Annu Rev Med* **48**: 283–293.

Tomlinson P, Sugarman ID (1995) Complications with shunts in adults with spina bifida. *BMJ* **311**: 286–287.

van Mechelen MC, Verhoef M, van Asbeck FWA, Post MW (2008) Work participation among young adults with spina bifida in the Netherlands. *Dev Med Child Neurol* **50**: 772–777.

Watson AR (2000) Non-compliance and transfer from paediatric to adult transplant unit. *Pediatr Nephrol* **14**: 469–472.

"Living Well" with Congenital Myasthenia: A Child and Family's Perspective

Gordon Webster, Kerry Webster, James Webster and Adam Webster

INTRODUCTION

There are several types of congenital myasthenic syndrome (CMS), an inherited neuromuscular disorder caused by different types of defect at the neuromuscular junction. Our family have a gene mutation that results in a deficiency of the acetylcholine receptors causing severe muscle weakness in all muscle groups. As babies/infants it caused feeding difficulties, respiratory problems, and resulted in a succession of hospital admissions.

The condition caused delays in the ability to sit, crawl and walk and for some of us in later life meant reliance on powered wheelchairs to aid with mobility. However, since three out of four of us have CMS, the condition has become part of our life and as a family we have never known life without it and we feel it has made us who we are.

DIAGNOSIS

Diagnosis of the condition has changed incredibly over the past 50 years since the first one of our family was diagnosed in the 1970s. At that time, it took more than 4 years for recognition that the severe weakness as an infant was due to myasthenia, and often, during this time, there were struggles to support healthy development of a child without a recognised medical condition. This involved lots of hospital admissions and visits to see the general practitioner (GP), as well as long nights and worries for both parents. By chance, a student doctor who had been studying myasthenia gravis noticed the child slumped in a chair with ptosis (drooping of the upper eyelid) and muscle weakness. A specific stay in hospital was then arranged to undertake a medical assessment, which included an intravenous neostigmine test (Tether 1948), and subsequently treatment with neostigmine tablets was commenced. However, despite the effectiveness of the medication in symptom management, this led to an incorrect diagnosis of myasthenia gravis, which stayed for the next 28 years until our first child was born. The diagnosis of CMS was never considered or thought of during these years despite muscle weakness being present from birth.

Diagnosis was different with the birth of our first child. Primary symptoms were again poor feeding, weak cry, and a failure to thrive, with repeated respiratory tract infections causing concern and necessitating many GP visits. After some initial assessments at the local hospital, we were taken to the nearby children's hospital where a Tensilon (edrophonium) test (Pascuzzi 2003) and successful treatment with pyridostigmine gave an initial diagnosis of CMS. A DNA blood test showed a mutation located within the acetylcholine receptor epsilon-subunit gene (Beeson et al. 2003) confirming a genetic diagnosis of CMS. When our child was 3 months old, we were referred to the National Specialised Congenital Myasthenia Service for further treatment.

Before the birth of our second child, we had genetic counselling, helping us understand that although most CMS is an autosomal recessive inherited disease, in our case (mother unaffected and father affected) we would have a 1:2 chance of another child with CMS. This was a chance worth taking as by now we were used to the condition and we knew that if it arose again we would be ready for its challenges. We therefore delayed knowing until after the birth even though we were offered early diagnosis through a prenatal blood test. This time the CMS diagnosis was within the first 2 weeks after birth. Diagnosis was quick because of availability of more routine testing for families with known CMS, similar to the gene screening they do now. Before the diagnosis, our second child then spent his first two weeks in an incubator, carefully monitored and fed through a nasogastric (NG) tube before pyridostigmine suspension could be given following the confirmed diagnosis.

EARLY LIFE WITH CONGENITAL MYASTHENIA

Medication (initially only pyridostigmine) was provided and this helped to some extent but weakness, illness and regular reviews and monitoring by health professionals became part of our daily life. We began to slowly adapt to emergency hospital admissions, long feeds and ensuring lots of rest periods and low levels of activity. Trying to limit activity for a toddler is challenging even if they have CMS. Walking was delayed until around 2 years, prior to this "bottom shuffling" was a favourite way of getting around. Food had to be pureed for a long time (even up to nursery). Choking was always a very real possibility, and there needed to be very careful management of medication, rest, eating and activity. The fluctuating nature of the weakness took a long time for others to understand. It was especially hard for people who did not live with CMS on a day-to-day basis to understand how tricky managing this condition was. Often plans had to be changed at the last moment and there was always a hospital bag packed and ready to go, which included relevant medical information and a care plan. We would have between 5 to 10 emergency hospital admissions each year. It was exhausting for the children, as lying down exacerbated the diaphragmatic weakness resulting in frequent coughs, snores and poor exhalation. This then caused tiredness in the day and increased levels of fatigue. It was often easier to support sleep by holding them in a sitting position; not much fun for the parent but helpful for the child as sleep was of a better quality.

Eating was problematic. There were often night feeds to catch up on those missed during the day. These broken nights not only affected the children but also impacted on the tiredness of the parent with CMS. Childhood illnesses also hit us hard and there were months when their health seemed to decline quickly. It was difficult to maintain sustained periods of wellness and daily activities were challenging. Despite all of this, development slowly continued and it was clear that we had clever, inquisitive and resilient children. As communication developed it was a lot easier to understand the levels of fatigue they were experiencing. Both children, by the time they started nursery school, had learned not to over exert themselves and to tell an adult when they needed rest.

ADAPTING TO LIFE WITH CONGENITAL MYASTHENIA

Over the years we have adapted to life with CMS. Taking life slowly and taking each day as it comes helps. We have learned to plan ahead and build in flexibility to manage fluctuating health needs. For example, when hospital visits were frequent we learned that not all medical staff were familiar with CMS (or myasthenia gravis) and it is very important to prepare a file on your child's needs. This file should include a letter from your GP/neurologist that enables you open access to a children's ward, avoiding a wait in the busy accident and emergency (A&E) department. Specific information on the type of CMS and how it affects your child, as well as copies of letters from recent appointments and lists of medications (including timings and dosages) are helpful for those supporting your child. It is also important to bring the medications with you and make staff aware that it is essential that they are administered on time. Always ask if you can be in charge of administering your child's medications, as hospital drug rounds do not always fit with your child's medication routine.

Since the boys are unable to use stairs and can only walk short distances, we moved to a bungalow, which was on one level, which could readily be modified and allow everyone to use all rooms. We have adapted the bathroom to a walk-in shower room equipped with a Clos-o-mat wash and dry toilet (http://www.clos-o-mat.com/) funded through a local authority Disabled Facilities Grant, which is not means tested for children under 19 years.

The boys use powered wheelchairs to aid mobility when outside of the home, provided by the local health service. This gives them independence and the ability to go places on their own. They both have had travel training provided through the local authority which enables them to use, unaccompanied, free public transport in the area with priority seating, allowing them to meet friends and socialise. Going to the cinema or concert is a favourable pastime as often a carer (or friend) can go free. These services may be different in other countries, but similar facilities need to be explored by parents.

CAREERS AND EDUCATION

Growing up with myasthenia in the 1970–1980s was difficult as no-one had heard of the condition and there was no school support. School friends could not understand absence from school and why sometimes I could play games at break and other times was too tired and had to stay indoors. Primary school was hard as I missed so much school time when younger from intercurrent illness. Because of this I remember not being able to read properly until the age of seven. However, my numeracy skills were good and because of an interest in the natural world, science became a hobby. High school science clubs were a good way of avoiding busy crowds at lunchtime. After continuing this interest at University, it led to a career in academia and scientific research which is perfect for someone with CMS as it allows flexible time management.

Today, getting the correct support for your child can still be a challenge as many professionals will have no experience of myasthenia and the fluctuating nature of the condition can result in others not recognising the impact of experiencing variable daily weakness. Education staff can be concerned about meeting complex health needs and require a lot of reassurance. We needed the help of doctors and nurses who knew the boys and how myasthenia affected them. We are so grateful for the support that the boys' medical team were able to provide, including talking to the school and attending annual reviews. Eventually both boys could access full-time support and mainstream school was accepted as the correct provision. Both boys use computers and read heavily, and presumably they will follow a career path that will suit their needs and interests especially with recent opportunities in information technology.

Recently, our eldest son James won a place at Oxford University to read Economics and this is what he has to say:

University is great fun with lots of opportunities to socialise. You can meet so many great people, and really delve into your chosen subject. University life will have its ups and downs but everyone will have their own challenges to overcome and if managing myasthenia will be one of yours then please read on. I found that sometimes I would feel too tired to go out, or the venue would not be accessible, so it may be difficult to socialise with some groups of people. That is OK, as the friends I did make clearly understood when I discussed my condition. Symptoms of myasthenia can fluctuate, and turning down invitations at the last minute can be hard or appear rude, but whenever I explained the situation, most people were very understanding. Academically, sometimes the work-load can be quite intense. Most universities offer extension periods if needed but this can be a slippery slope as you always have to catch up. To stay on top, I would try to get a decent number of hours of sleep and then do most of my work in the mornings when I felt strongest. This would leave evenings free for meeting friends. I needed more help with laundry but I chose a college accommodation where evening meals were provided, and for breakfast/lunch I became very good at using the microwave. I had help to get library books and because of my CMS (special circumstance), I would get an extension to keep books out for as long as I needed them.

Before I went to University, I was assessed for a disability student's grant [https://www.gov.uk/ disabled-students-allowances-dsas]. This allowed me to purchase a laptop, printer and Dictaphone. If I could not make any lectures due to illness, then someone would go and record them. So much can now be done electronically that I did not feel that I was at a disadvantage. Sometimes the tutorials were held in my room and this made it really easy. I was also able to complete all my exams in a small room on the college site with extra time provided if needed. I was allocated an accessible room and stayed in the same room for the 3 years, which again was a great help. I recommend talking to the university officers; do not be worried to ask for what you need. Everyone was always happy to help.

MEDICATIONS

Over the course of the last 20 years the boys' medications have changed and this has had a huge impact on the weakness they experience. In 2014, a new medication Salbutamol/Albuterol (Rodríguez Cruz et al. 2015) was introduced that enabled the boys to walk and become much more independent, including participating in wheelchair Karate competitions. It was so important that we were able to access the specialist neuromuscular clinics to allow this change to be introduced. At some points in the past, we have had to use non-invasive ventilation, oxygen and suction at home and to be trained in cardio-pulmonary resuscitation (CPR). Luckily, this is no longer the case and despite managing severe weakness for a long time there is always hope that new treatments can bring improvement.

BENEFITS AND ENTITLEMENTS

Ask about what will help financially and practically. We have been supported through the benefits system and the boys have received Disability Living Allowance and Personal Independence Payment. The boys have had additional support in school through the additional needs assessment process and they were transported to and from school. We have adapted our home with the support of a disabled facilities grant. The boys have also accessed opportunities to travel and to develop their independence skills through Dream Flight and Whizz Kids.

HELPFUL TIPS

- Having a good medical team that know you and your child.
- Keep a file of all important information so that others can learn about CMS and how it affects the individual concerned.

- Organise medications and use pharmacy delivery services where possible. Put dates in your diary when you need to re-order medications. Allow your child to be as independent as possible when taking medication.
- Be proactive and plan for transitions in school. Make sure there is a robust healthcare plan and all adults have an understanding of the fluctuating nature of weakness. Be patient and positive with those who have a helping role – they will not have your understanding or experience of supporting. Help them to help you.
- A home–school book is useful to record changes in levels of fatigue, times of medications and issues arising during the school day. Note that this book is useful to alert teachers when the child has had a poor night's sleep or is under the weather.
- Develop a script for your child so they can share what myasthenia is and support how they communicate their weakness to other people.
- Once all your basic needs have been met, such as sleep, diet and movement, then be as adventurous as you can. Know your limits but don't limit yourself. Myasthenia is only part of what your family and life is about.
- Pace yourself, do what you can when you can and leave the other stuff for a stronger day.
- Ask for help; access the support from Myaware and other relevant charities.
- Look after yourself and exercise, whilst this may be limited by muscle weakness and fatigue, take as much exercise as possible. Physiotherapy can help as this prevents complications, such as joint contractures (stiffness).
- If you are a carer, you also need to be in good shape to be able to provide care. Make sure you look after your needs and seek help when needed.

SOME ADVICE FOR FAMILIES AND SCHOOLS

These are some simple tips to help children with CMS at school, although they are equally applicable to life at home. You may wish to discuss them with the specialist educational needs coordinator (SENCO) in school.

- Use a chair of suitable height to sit comfortably at a desk. Avoid sitting on the floor to prevent having to get up and down frequently.
- Make the school aware that it is essential that your child needs to take their medications on time and without fail. A record of medications times should be used to prevent mistakes or record forgotten or late medication doses.
- Ensure extra time for completing exercise work, tests and exams.
- Use a computer or laptop instead of writing.
- An agreed Education and Health Care Plan (EHCP) is often needed to get extra assistance, equipment and help in the school. This plan will also help with obtaining school transport.
- Try not to avoid physical education (PE) within the school curriculum, but discuss whether and how much your child should join in PE and sport lessons. Make the school aware of the child's limitations.
- When tired, your child should be allowed to stay indoors during playtime. Alternatively, a quiet seated area in the playground may also be useful.
- Allow for starting late and leaving early.
- Avoid having to stand in queues.
- Make teachers aware that a child with CMS cannot always raise a hand to be noticed or increase their voice to be heard.

- Explain to the school and friends about CMS and the difficulties associated with it. If you are not confident with this, a health professional (e.g. school nurse) will gladly help.
- Caring adults need to be aware of signs of weakness to remind the child to rest. Symptoms of CMS typically vary from day to day and time to time and therefore a child may appear strong one day and not the next.
- At meal times, allow enough time to eat a meal or drink a drink safely and slowly.
- Sometimes the symptoms of CMS (e.g. ptosis, squint, slurred speech and low speech volume) can make the child appear different. This can result in unkind comments and should be treated sensitively by all adults.
- Adequate disabled toilet facilities should be put in place.
- Referral to the community paediatricians and community paediatric nursing teams are important sources of advice and support.
- In addition to routine vaccinations, children and adults with CMS should have a flu vaccine every year. They should also consider the pneumococcal vaccine (e.g. Prevnar), if they have not had it as part of routine immunisation schedule.
- Your child should be encouraged and helped to lead as normal a life as possible. Sensible precautions and interventions should be adopted – try not to go over-board.

USEFUL WEBSITES

Myaware

https://www.myaware.org/

A United Kingdom charity dedicated solely to the care and support of people affected by myasthenia.

CONTACT

https://contact.org.uk/

United Kingdom charity that supports families with disabled children offering the best possible guidance and information.

IPSEA (Independent provider of special education advice)

https://www.ipsea.org.uk/

IPSEA is a registered charity operating in England offering free and independent legally based information, advice and support to help get the right education for children and young people with all kinds of special educational needs and disabilities (SEND). They also provide training on SEND legal framework to parents and carers.

Working Families

https://www.workingfamilies.org.uk/

This society offers advice in balancing the demands of family and work at different life stages. It also has a special section, titled the Waving Not Drowning Network, that has a helpline, Facebook page, newsletter, e-bulletin, events and publications for parents of disabled children.

Rare Disease UK

https://www.raredisease.org.uk/

Rare Disease UK (RDUK) is a national campaign for people with rare diseases. RDUK provides a voice for the rare disease community by sharing the experiences of patients and families.

Personal Independence Payment (PIP)

https://www.gov.uk/pip

Financial help for long-term ill-health or disability.

Disabled Facilities Grants

https://www.gov.uk/disabled-facilities-grants

Grant available from your council if you are disabled and need to make changes to your home.

REFERENCES

Beeson D, Webster R, Ealing J et al. (2003) Structural abnormalities of the AChR caused by mutations underlying congenital myasthenic syndromes. *Ann N Y Acad Sci* **998:** 114–124.

Pascuzzi RM (2003) The edrophonium test. *Seminars in Neurology* **23:** 83–88.

Rodríguez Cruz PM, Palace JD, Ramjattan H, Jayawant S, Robb SA, Beeson D (2015) Salbutamol and ephedrine in the treatment of severe AChR deficiency syndromes. *Neurology* **85:** 1043–1047.

Tether JE (1948) Intravenous neostigmine in diagnosis of myasthenia gravis. *Ann Intern Med* **29:** 1132–1138.

Index

More titles from Mac Keith Press www.mackeith.co.uk

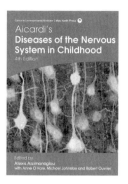

Aicardi's Diseases of the Nervous System in Childhood, 4th Edition

Alexis Arzimanoglou with Anne O'Hare, Michael V Johnston and Robert Ouvrier (Editors)

Clinics in Developmental Medicine
2018 ▪ 1524pp ▪ hardback ▪ 78-1-909962-80-4

This fourth edition retains the patient-focussed, clinical approach of its predecessors. The international team of editors and contributors has honoured the request of the late Jean Aicardi, that his book remain 'resolutely clinical', which distinguishes *Diseases of the Nervous System in Childhood* from other texts in the field. New edition completely updated and revised and now in full colour.

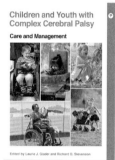

Children and Youth with Complex Cerebral Palsy: Care and Management

Laurie J. Glader and Richard D. Stevenson (Editors)

A practical guide from Mac Keith Press
2019 ▪ 404pp ▪ softback ▪ 978-1-909962-98-9

This is the first practical guide to explore management of the many medical comorbidities that children with complex CP face, including orthopaedics, mobility needs, cognition and sensory impairment, difficult behaviours, respiratory complications and nutrition, amongst others. Uniquely, contributors include children and parents, providing applied wisdom for family-centred care. Clinical Care Tools are provided to help guide clinicians and include a Medical Review Supplement, Equipment and Services Checklist and an ICF-Based Care: Goals and Management Form.

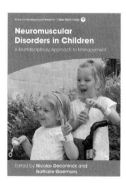

Neuromuscular Disorders in Children: A Multidisciplinary Approach to Management

Nicolas Deconinck and Nathalie Goemans (Editors)

Clinics in Developmental Medicine
2019 ▪ 468pp ▪ hardback ▪ 978-1-911612-08-7

This book critically reviews current evidence of management approaches in the field of neuromuscular disorders in children. Uniquely, the book focusses on assessment as the cornerstone of management and highlights the importance of a multidisciplinary approach.

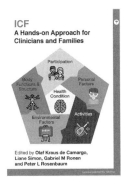

ICF: A Hands-on Approach for Clinicians and Families

Olaf Kraus de Camargo, Liane Simon, Gabriel M. Ronen and Peter L. Rosenbaum (Editors)

A practical guide from Mac Keith Press
2019 ▪ 192pp ▪ softback ▪ 978-1-911612-04-9

This accessible handbook introduces the World Health Organisation's International Classification of Functioning, Disability and Health (ICF) to professionals working with children with disabilities and their families. It contains an overview of the elements of the ICF but focusses on practical applications, including how the ICF framework can be used with children, families and carers to formulate health and management goals.

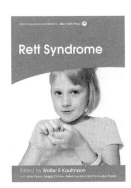

Rett Syndrome

Walter E Kaufmann, Alan Percy, Angus Clarke, Helen Leonard and SakkuBai Naidu (Editors)

Clinics in Developmental Medicine
2017 ▪ 240pp ▪ hardback ▪ 978-1-909962-83-5

Among the vast body of literature that has grown around Rett syndrome, this volume is the first to be aimed at both clinicians and researchers. It presents a comprehensive overview of the disorder and examines the areas where gaps in knowledge are most significant. *Rett Syndrome* is intended to be a guide for both initial examination and in-depth study of the disorder. It is a practical text for the physician approaching the disorder for the first time and a valuable reference resource for the specialist or researcher.

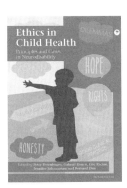

Ethics in Child Health:
Principles and Cases in Neurodisability

Peter L Rosenbaum, Gabriel M Ronen, Eric Racine, Jennifer Johannesen and Bernard Dan (Editors)

A practical guide from Mac Keith Press
2016 ▪ 384pp ▪ softback ▪ 978-1-909962-63-7

Ethics in Child Health offers a set of principles that clinicians, social workers and policy-makers can utilise in their respective spheres of influence. Each chapter is built around a scenario familiar to clinicians and is discussed with respect to how ethical principles can be utilised to inform decision-making. Useful 'Themes for Discussion' are provided at the end of each chapter to help professionals and students develop practical ethical thinking.

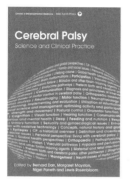

Cerebral Palsy: Science and Clinical Practice
Bernard Dan, Margaret Mayston, Nigel Paneth and Lewis Rosenbloom (Editors)

Clinics in Developmental Medicine
2015 ▪ 648pp ▪ hardback ▪ 978-1-909962-38-5

This landmark title considers all aspects of cerebral palsy from the causes to clinical problems and their implications for individuals. An international team of experts present a wide range of person-centred assessment approaches, including clinical evaluation, measurement scales, neuroimaging and gait analysis. The perspective of the book spans the lifelong course of cerebral palsy, taking into account worldwide differences in socio-economic and cultural factors. Full integrated colour, with extensive cross-referencing make this a highly attractive and useful reference.

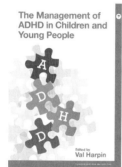

The Management of ADHD in Children and Young People
Val Harpin (Editor)

A practical guide from Mac Keith Press
2017 ▪ 292pp ▪ softback ▪ 978-1-909962-72-9

This book is an accessible and practical guide on all aspects of assessment of children and young people with Attention Deficit Hyperactivity Disorder (ADHD) and how they can be managed successfully. The multi-professional team of authors discusses referral, assessment and diagnosis, psychological management, pharmacological management, and co-existing conditions, as well as ADHD in the school setting. New research on girls with ADHD is also featured. Case scenarios are included that bring these topics to life.

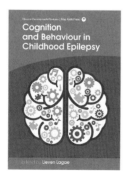

Cognition and Behaviour in Childhood Epilepsy
Lieven Lagae (Editor)

Clinics in Developmental Medicine
2017 ▪ 186pp ▪ hardback ▪ 978-1-909962-87-3

For many parents, cognitive and behavioral comorbidities, such as ADHD, autism and intellectual disability, are the real burden of childhood epilepsy. This title offers concrete guidance and treatment strategies for childhood epilepsy in general, and for the comorbidities associated with each epilepsy syndrome and their pathophysiology. The book is written by experts in the field with an important clinical experience, while chapters by clinical neuropsychologists provide a strong theoretical background.

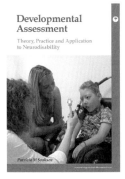

Developmental Assessment: Theory, Practice and Application to Neurodisability
Patricia M. Sonksen

A practical guide from Mac Keith Press
2016 ▪ 384pp ▪ softback ▪ 978-1-909962-56-9

This handbook presents a new approach to assessing development in preschool children that can be applied across the developmental spectrum. The reader is taught how to confirm whether development is typical, and if it is not, is signposted to the likely nature and severity of the impairments with a plan of action. The author uses numerous case vignettes from her 40 years' experience to bring to life her approach with clear summary key points and helpful illustrations.

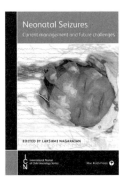

Neonatal Seizures:
Current Management and Future Challenges
Lakshmi Nagarajan (Editor)

International Reviews of Child Neurology
2016 ▪ 214pp ▪ hardback ▪978-1-909962-67-5

A better understanding of neural activity and the development of cortical connections and networks is an important requirement for evaluating the cause and treatment of neonatal seizures. There have been many advances in the management of neonatal seizures such as increased use of EEGs, therapeutic hypothermia for HIE and exome sequencing, to name a few. This book distils what is known about these advances into one scholarly yet practical text.

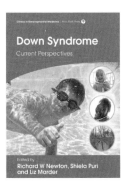

Down Syndrome: Current Perspectives
Richard W. Newton, Shiela Puri and Liz Marder (Editors)

Clinics in Developmental Medicine
2015 ▪ 320pp ▪ hardback ▪ 978-1-909962-47-7

Down syndrome remains the most common recognisable form of intellectual disability. The challenge for doctors today is how to capture the rapidly expanding body of scientific knowledge and devise models of care to meet the needs of individuals and their families. *Down Syndrome: Current Perspectives* provides doctors and other health professionals with the information they need to address the challenges that can present in the management of this syndrome.